A Technician's Guide
to Exotic Animal Care

A Technician's Guide
to Exotic Animal Care

Thomas N. Tully, Jr., DVM, MS
Diplomate ABVP (avian)
Associate Professor
Department Veterinary Clinical Sciences
Louisiana State University–School of Veterinary Medicine
Baton Rouge, Louisiana, USA

Mark A. Mitchell, DVM, MS
Assistant Professor
Department Veterinary Clinical Sciences
Louisiana State University–School of Veterinary Medicine
Baton Rouge, Louisiana, USA

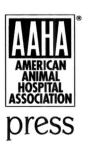

AAHA®
AMERICAN
ANIMAL
HOSPITAL
ASSOCIATION
press

Many thanks to the Learning and Development Advisory Group
Dr. Laurel Collins, ABVP
Dr. Richard Goebel
Dr. Charles Hickey
Dr. Clayton McKinnon
Dr. Hal Taylor

Edited by Susan K. Fedel

Book and cover design by Carolyn Cork Rech

American Animal Hospital Association
AAHA Press
12575 West Bayaud Avenue
Lakewood, Colorado 80228

Printed in the United States of America
10 9 8 7 6 5 4 3 2 1

ISBN 1-58326-012-9

        Library of Congress Cataloging-in-Publication Data
Tully, Thomas N.
  A technician's guide to exotic animal care /
  Thomas N. Tully, Jr., Mark A. Mitchell
        p. cm.
  Includes bibliographical references (p.).
  ISBN 1-58326-012-9
  1. Exotic animals–Diseases. 2. Wildlife diseases. 3. Pet medicine. 4. Veterinary
nursing. I. Mitchell, Mark A., 1967- II. Title.

SF997.5.E95 T85 2001
636.089'073–dc21
                                                    2001022120
                                                    CIP

Contents

CHAPTER 3

FERRETS 81

ILLUSTRATIONS

Chapter 1–AVIAN

Figure 1-1 A typical outdoor flight. This is a raised outdoor flight for medium-sized parrots with nest boxes visible in the background.

Figure 1-2 A Plexiglas® cage. Plexiglas® cages are one of the many new cage designs that enhance a bird's presence in the house. This type of cage also prevents debris and feathers from falling to the floor.

Figure 1-3 Pelleted diet. Advances in avian nutrition have led to the development of more nutritious pelleted diets for many species of pet birds.

Figure 1-4 Sipper bottle. These bottles are recommended to prevent fecal contamination of the water supply.

Figure 1-5 A Cuttlebone is shown with other calcium supplements for pet birds. Cuttlebones do not sharpen the beak, but provide a source of nutritional calcium.

Figure 1-6 Pet carrier. Carriers are recommended for transport of small and large pet birds.

Figure 1-7 The proper holding method for small cage birds.

Figure 1-8 Grasping a bird around the neck using an Elizabethan grip.

Figure 1-9 Proper technique to hold a large pet bird.

Figure 1-10 An avian restraint board with bird in it. Avian restraint boards adequately restrain birds for physical examinations, diagnostics, sampling, and radiology.

Figure 1-11 Commercial beak speculums for small and large bird species.

Figure 1-12 Normal keel versus thin keel. Pectoral musculature helps determine the body condition of an avian patient. A full-bodied bird with a well-developed pectoral muscle mass usually indicates good health.

Figure 1-13 The uropygial gland is located at the caudal dorsal aspect of any avian species. This gland aids in feather grooming and waterproofing. It is very well developed in aquatic avian species.

Figure 1-14 One-handed blood draw. Proper technique is being used in drawing blood from the right jugular vein.

Figure 1-15 Microtainer® tubes. This is a typical 0.5ml blood collection tube used in avian diagnostic testing.

Figure 1-16 Proximal tibiotarsal bone. This is the site of choice for bone marrow aspiration.

Figure 1-17 Scaly face mites. The white areas involving the edges of the upper beak and lower beak are consistent with hyperkeritosis. This condition is attributed to scaly face mite infestation and is commonly seen in budgerigars.

Figure 1-18 A Dremel® tool shown with other nail trimming accessories. A handheld, motor-driven tool is commonly used to groom beaks and trim toenails of larger pet birds.

Figure 1-19 Flight feathers. The pointer is showing the primary flight feathers, which are commonly trimmed to restrict the pet bird's flight.

Figure 1-20 Blood feathers. Growing flight feathers are often called blood feathers because the ensheathed, developing feather is nourished by a significant blood supply.

Chapter 2–REPTILES AND AMPHIBIANS

Chapter 3–FERRETS

Figure 3-1 Albino ferret. The distinguishing characteristics of an albino ferret are its white coat and pink eyes.

Figure 3-2 A sable ferret is identified by distinctive black markings on his face and body.

Figure 3-3 An example of a typical history form that can be used to evaluate a ferret's health.

Figure 3-4 "Scruffing" a ferret. Although grabbing a ferret by the nape appears traumatic, it is actually the preferred method of holding a ferret to perform a physical examination.

Figure 3-5 Alopecia. Ferrets can develop a generalized hair loss due to a number of disease processes. The most common disease presentation in which generalized hair loss occurs is adrenal disease.

Figure 3-6 Swollen ferret vulva. The swollen vulva, which may occur due to hormonal influence, can become very prominent.

Figure 3-7 Anterior vena cava venipuncture. Blood collection utilizing the anterior vena cava provides ready access to large volumes of blood.

Figure 3-8 Technique used for blood collection from the cephalic vein of a ferret.

Figure 3-9 Technique used for blood collection from the lateral saphenous vein of a ferret.

Figure 3-10 "Masking down." Ferret anesthetic induction is achieved through an induction chamber or a facemask (as shown).

Figure 3-11 Insulinoma. Notice the neoplastic nodule within the pancreas.

Figure 3-12 Lymphoma. Notice the enlarged mesenteric lymph node.

Chapter 4–RABBITS

Figure 4-1A Typical outdoor housing for pet rabbits. The cage protects the rabbit from predators and inclement weather.

Figure 4-1B Morant pen. This outdoor hutch allows the rabbit access to the sun and grass, while providing shelter in the event of a storm.

Figure 4-1C Indoor rabbit housing. This pop-up style rabbit hutch has a place for food and a water bottle.

Figure 4-2 Typical sipper water bottle. This type of bottle is recommended for rabbit enclosures.

Figure 4-3A A New Zealand White. These rabbits have been popular pets and have been used in laboratory studies for many years.

Figure 4-3B A Netherlands Dwarf. This rabbit, which is being properly held, can be identified by its small body conformation and ears.

Figure 4-4 Proper holding. A rabbit should be properly held on the exam table by grabbing the scruff of the neck and supporting the rear legs.

Figure 4-5A Frontal view.

Figure 4-5B Side view. A bunny burrito is another form of rabbit restraint that utilizes a towel to prevent excess leg movement.

Figure 4-6 Proper technique to transport a rabbit. Make sure that the rabbit's rear legs are supported as the opposite hand has a firm grip on the scruff of the neck.

Chapter 5–RODENTS

Chapter 6–HEDGEHOGS

Figure 6-1A Hedgehogs are covered in spines.

Figure 6-1B Hedgehogs, however, do not have spines on their faces or abdomens.

Figure 6-2 Oral mass. Tumors are often seen in pet hedgehogs.

Chapter 7–SUGAR GLIDERS

Figure 7-1 Sugar gliders are small marsupials native to Australia and New Guinea.

Figure 7-2 A female sugar glider is shown here with her young.

Figure 7-3 Sugar glider food. Manufactured food is available to prevent common health problems associated with malnutrition.

Chapter 8–FISH

Figure 8-1 Fish food. A variety of food used for fish maintained in hobby aquariums is shown here.

Figure 8-2 Power filter. This is a typical external filter used in hobby fish aquariums.

Figure 8-3 Test kit. Kits such as the one shown here are needed to determine and maintain water quality in aquariums.

Figure 8-4 Hands-on examination. The proper way to hold a fish for a complete physical exam is shown here.

Figure 8-5 Gill biopsy. This is a useful diagnostic tool for identifying diseases associated with the gills.

Figure 8-6 Skin scrape. Common skin pathogens are identified through skin scraping and microscopic examination.

Figure 8-7 Fin biopsy. Certain disease processes may be identified through a fin biopsy.

Figure 8-8 Venipuncture. The most useful vein for blood collection in fish is the caudal tail vein.

Figure 8-9 Therapeutics. Proper position is shown for intraperitoneal injection.

Figure 8-10 Force-feeding. Medication and feeding through a tube is necessary in debilitated fish patients.

Figure 8-11 *Ichthyopthirius multifiliis.* Shown is a microscopic view of the *Ich.* organism.

Figure 8-12 *Saprolegnia.* Shown is a microscopic view of the *Sapro.* organism.

TABLES

Chapter 1–AVIAN

Chapter 2–REPTILES AND AMPHIBIANS

Chapter 3–FERRETS

Chapter 4–RABBITS

Chapter 5–RODENTS

Chapter 6–HEDGEHOGS

Chapter 7–SUGAR GLIDERS

PREFACE

Companion exotic animals encompass a wide variety of species that include birds, reptiles, ferrets, rabbits, rodents, hedgehogs, small marsupials, and fish. With this wide variety of animals, there are a growing number of owners who seek veterinary care for their exotic pets. These owners are looking for quality care, and they expect technicians and veterinarians to have basic knowledge of handling, diseases, husbandry, and nutrition. However, with the number of species within the exotic animal classification, it may seem impossible to gain the experience needed to feel comfortable treating and handling these unique patients. This text provides the essential information in a systematic formula that covers the basic responsibilities of veterinary technicians. Exotic companion animal owners should be encouraged to seek veterinary care for their animals when first purchased and, at least, on a yearly basis for health examinations. The initial visit helps prevent one of the most common causes of death in pet exotic animals: improper care/nutrition. Examination of the patient and, more importantly, education of the owner are the primary objectives of the first visit. The education process can incorporate discussion, handouts, videotapes, and recommended Internet Web sites.

Veterinarians need and actively seek technicians who have an interest and expertise in working with exotic animal species. To gain this needed experience one must initially have the interest to become experienced in handling and collecting diagnostic samples from these animals. The basic knowledge learned on dogs and cats will serve the interested exotic animal veterinary technician well, and confidence will quickly grow in proportion to the number of animals treated. Each chapter covers the following main topics: husbandry, nutrition, restraint, physical examination, and diagnostic sampling, therapeutics, and diseases. There are references at the end of each chapter for individuals who seek more detailed information on a particular topic. For the majority of veterinary technicians, this book will provide the basic guidance to perform quality pet care. As stated earlier, an increasing number of people own exotic companion animals, and veterinarians want interested/qualified technicians to help meet this need. The authors encourage veterinary technicians to get involved in this exciting and challenging section of veterinary medicine.

ACKNOWLEDGMENTS

The authors gratefully acknowledge the help and assistance of Ms. Mary-Claire Holley, Ms. Lisa Peri, Mr. Harry Cowgill, Mr. Micheal Broussard, and Ms. Nancy Loupe. Their work was essential to the successful completion of this text.

The moral support and ability to put up with the authors' constant emotional demands while working on this project was provided by Susie Tully, Claudia Rose Tully, and Lorrie Hale-Mitchell. The authors dedicate this book to them.

CHAPTER 1

AVIAN

INTRODUCTION

There are close to 9,000 different avian species worldwide. These are not different breeds of the same species, like dogs and cats, but are, in fact, entirely different animals within the class Aves. When someone first comprehends this difference, it would seem that it is impossible to become qualified to treat so many different types of birds. With this in mind, a technician must learn and become knowledgeable about basic avian husbandry, diagnostic sampling, and patient care. Most veterinary practices see only companion avian species (e.g., parrots, macaws and cockatiels) and caged birds (e.g., finches and canaries). These are the species that technicians need to become familiar with and comfortable handling and treating. Through experience and modification of technical skills, the transition between avian species is easy to make, if needed, for wildlife or zoological avian species (e.g., toucans, flamingos, penguins, or ostriches). Companion avian species need to be examined yearly, groomed regularly, and vaccinated on a regular schedule. As with other exotic species, the presentation of the patient in the exam room allows the technician to provide husbandry and nutritional information to the client. Captive-reared companion avian species are excellent pets, with each species having advantages and disadvantages to ownership—similar to the physical and personality differences observed in cat and dog breeds. If placed on a proper diet and maintained on that nutritional regimen for their entire life, most pet birds are provided the nutrition to live long, healthy lives.

HUSBANDRY

ENVIRONMENTAL CONCERNS

Most new pet bird owners purchase their pets with a few preconceived ideas that have been learned from a lifetime of hearing misinformation. One is that birds are sensitive to cold and drafts. In reality, avian species are much more sensitive to heat than cold and/or drafts. Birds have an ability to acclimatize to almost any environment over time, especially cooler weather. Although many birds come from arid, tropical, and subtropical regions of the world, there are microenvironments within these areas that provide protection from the oppressive heat. Many of these microenvironments range from 75–85°F. If parrots are allowed to stay outside in a protected cage against the prevailing wind with a roof and nest box, they will acclimatize to temperatures that drop into the lower 30°F range (Figure 1-1). Temperatures that drop lower than freezing will require the owner to place a heat lamp for temperature regulation. Birds will respond to indoor temperatures much the same as they do to outside seasonal variations. They will molt feathers in the spring as the hotter summer months approach, and molt and produce more down feathers in the autumn as the cooler winter months approach. Although owners may complain about the extra feather loss in the spring and autumn, this is not an unusual finding. Even with air conditioning, the ambient temperature of the house rises and falls with the position of the cage and season of the year. It is not recommended to move a bird that has been housed in an air-conditioned environment into an outdoor flight during the peak months of summer or winter because they are not acclimatized to the environment. Added stress may come from placing a bird under/over a vent from the air-conditioning system since this air is

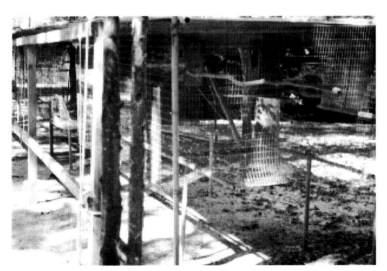

Figure 1-1 A typical outdoor flight. This is a raised outdoor flight for medium-sized parrots with nest boxes visible in the background.

considerably cooler/warmer than the surrounding air temperature. The problem that develops from this location is added physical stress on the bird to compensate for the constant change in temperature as the system shuts off and on to maintain the thermostat setting. It is recommended to place the cage in a room in which there is interaction with the other family members, away from direct vent airflow.

Cage design has been elevated to an art. There are many different cage designs manufactured from different products, ranging from brass wire to Plexiglas® (Figure 1-2). Most cage designs are for indoor use only, and it is recommended that most, if not all, commercial cages be used only indoors. Owners who buy the cage for indoor use usually do so based on individual taste and the interior design of their house. The only requirement from a health point of view is that the cage be of appropriate size for the bird(s) being maintained in the structure. This also includes the addition of perches and toys. There has been a tendency for owners to "love their birds too much" by adding too many perches and toys. An abundance of these items increases the chance for injury and does not provide adequate exercise space. Perches and toys should be appropriate for the bird's size. Budgerigar toys and perches are inappropriate for an Amazon Parrot. Natural wood perches, cut from hardwood trees (e.g., oak,

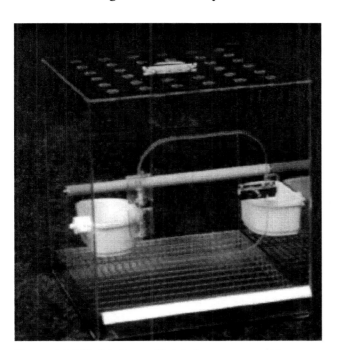

Figure 1-2 A Plexiglas® cage. Plexiglas® cages are one of the many new cage designs that enhance a bird's presence in the house. This type of cage also prevents debris and feathers from falling to the floor.

maple, or hickory) are recommended for pet birds. The natural wood can be readily replaced, and it also provides a variable diameter and foot surface for the birds to use, which helps to exercise the feet. Never use sandpaper on the perches because this causes irritation to the foot area that comes into contact with this abrasive surface.

Newspaper is the substrate of choice to line the cage bottom. This substrate is cheap and allows the owner to observe the fecal material from the bird, thereby monitoring the eating habits and gastrointestinal system of his pet. Newspaper also gets dirty, making it readily apparent to the owner that routine cleaning of the cage is required. Other substances (e.g., ground walnut shells and corncobs) used as birdcage substrate dry out fecal material and hide excreta from the owner, giving him the impression that the cage is "clean;" there have been instances of birds ingesting this material. The majority of pet birds maintained inside do not need grit to aid in food digestion. These birds shell their seed and, for the most part, grind the kernel, forgoing the need for grit. If an owner insists on using grit, crushed oyster shell or egg shell is recommended as not only a mechanical means to grind the food in the ventriculus, but also as a dietary calcium source. The anti-mite tin that contains an insecticide disk to be placed on the outside of the cage is also not recommended. Pet birds that are housed inside do not come into contact with lice or mites, and the insecticide will not affect the mites that are commonly diagnosed infesting budgerigars. Sandpaper perches, grit, and anti-mite devices are a waste of money for pet bird owners and, in many cases, will contribute to health problems.

Outdoor flights are uniformly manufactured through private companies or owners using different gauges of hardware cloth and J-clips. The outdoor flights are built according to the bird's size and the breeding requirements of that particular species. The main requirements for outdoor flights are: appropriate size and wire gauge, flight maintained off the ground, proper nest box structure, roof or partial roof, prevailing wind protection (especially in the winter), and heat lamp when applicable. Predator control is essential in outdoor flights and large aviary buildings, since there have been a number of tragic cases of predators (especially raccoons) attacking birds housed outdoors. In addition, opossums can excrete a parasite in their feces, *Sarcocystis* spp., which is then eaten by cockroaches and deposited (by way of feces) in the bird food. It is also very difficult, but vital, to control vermin and insects in complex aviary structures, because these pests can carry a number of bacterial and parasitic diseases. Any predator, insect, and/or vermin control program must take into account bird exposure to the agent being used for eradication of these pests.

NUTRITION

This area of companion avian medicine has been one of the most active in advancing the health of companion birds. Twenty years ago the only commercially available feed was seed for parrots. Of course, if an owner has another species of bird (e.g., pigeons, peafowl, waterfowl, and ratites), the commercially available feed is recommended.

For companion avian species, which include parrots, macaws, and caged songbirds, advances have been made in the form of pellets (Figure 1-3). These pelleted bird diets are manufactured by a number of companies and come in many shapes, sizes, and tastes. The secret to getting a bird transitioned from a seed diet to a pelleted diet is to start young and, if possible, to allow the bird to see other birds eating the pellets. If the pellets are colored, some birds will eat only specific colors and this may change the color of the fecal material. This does not cause any health problems, but does assure the owner that the bird is eating the pellets and not just crushing them in the beak. Although some feed manufacturers promote pelleted diets as containing all of the needed nutrients for a complete diet, a diversified diet with pellets as the foundation is recommended. This diversified diet should contain seeds, vegetables, possibly cheese and cooked eggs, and a small amount of fruit. Some pet bird species, which have fruit as a large part of their diet, (such as Lories) require a greater percentage of fruit and nectar. As always, it is up to the owner to research the nutritional requirements of his pet and make sure that the proper diet is provided. The diversified diet not only supplements a variety of nutritional components, but also psychologically stimulates the bird with different

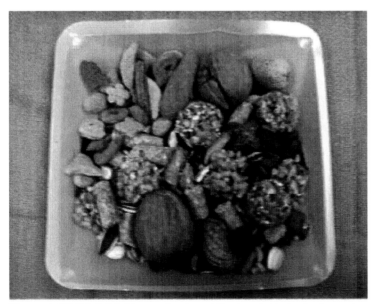

Figure 1-3 Pelleted diet. Advances in avian nutrition have led to the development of more nutritious pelleted diets for many species of pet birds.

sizes and textures of the foodstuffs that it eats. A psychologically stimulated bird is a happy bird that may exhibit reduced vices, such as feather picking, and stimulated reproductive activity.

Fresh water should always be available. The water container should be cleaned daily and refilled with a fresh supply. To prevent "poop soup," sipper bottles that attach to the side of the cage are recommended for parrot species (Figure 1-4). The birds cannot dump the container in the bottom of the cage or defecate in their water. The bird's beak and tongue should be touched to the tip of the sipper tube when first introduced to make sure the animal knows that water is available at the end of this strange stainless steel device.

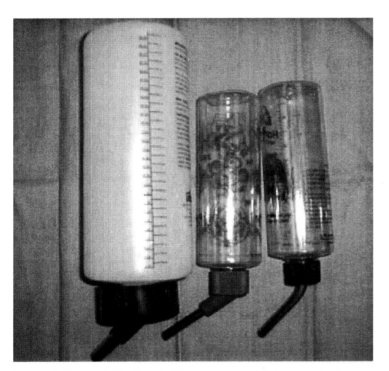

Figure 1-4 Sipper bottle. These bottles are recommended to prevent fecal contamination of the water supply.

Stick treats can be provided, but the stick and wire need to be removed from the cage once the bird has finished eating the attached seeds. Spray millet, millet on the natural seed head, is a welcome treat to smaller psittacine species, such as lovebirds and cockatiels.

Calcium supplementation is a must, and for smaller birds, a cuttlebone will provide the source (Figure 1-5). The soft side faces the bird and the bird eats the bone, as calcium is required in the diet. These are not beak-sharpening devices, but calcium sources. For larger birds, a mineral block will provide the calcium supplement, because they can crush a cuttlebone in seconds. If an owner wants to place a vitamin and/or mineral supplement in the water or on the bird's food, he must strictly follow the

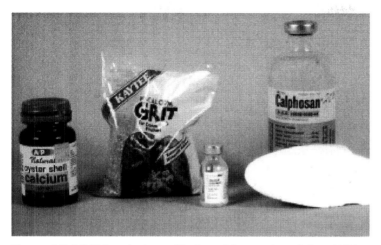

Figure 1-5 A Cuttlebone is shown with other calcium supplements for pet birds. Cuttlebones do not sharpen the beak, but provide a source of nutritional calcium.

instructions provided with that product. Often, birds will not drink or eat substances that have been tainted, which can reduce the required nutritional intake of these pets. If the bird does drink the water and eat the food with the supplement, both containers need to be cleaned daily because of vitamin degradation and predisposition to bacterial growth.

HISTORY

As with other animal species, it is very important to get a thorough history from the owner prior to examining the avian patient. Identification is the first important information that the examiner needs to obtain from the owner. Identification includes the name of the patient, species of bird, and the age (if known). Birds can be obtained from a number of sources, so it is important to know how long the animal has been at that particular house and where it was acquired in order to determine the overall patient health. Find out whether the owner can provide a vaccination history, when the bird last molted, and the character of feces. Most birds coming into the clinic will be companion animals, but some are breeding birds that are seldom, if ever, handled. Ask the owner if the bird is a pet bird or a breeding bird and how often it is taken out of the cage. Most breeding birds are housed in outdoor flights, but a specific understanding of where the bird is maintained is needed to determine if there has been any possible exposure to wild avian species or vermin. Since most owners will bring the patient in plastic pet carriers, the history should include the type and size of cage, substrate, toys and perches, disinfectants used, and regularity of cleaning the cage (Figure 1-6).

Once the environment has been determined, nutrition is the next major area of questioning. The specific brand, type and amount of food, as well as how much the bird eats on a daily basis (prior to the presenting problem and since it has been ill) must be determined. If there are any supplements or treats offered, a notation should be made on the form. How often the water is changed and the source of the water may be useful questions to ask the owner. There have been published cases of embryonic and neonatal deaths that were caused by well water and automatic watering systems that contained bacteria.

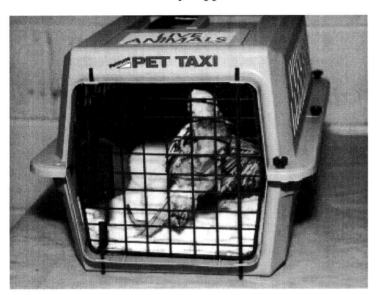

Figure 1-6 Pet carrier. Carriers are recommended for transport of small and large pet birds.

A review of the total pet household, including other birds, must be noted in the history. This information would incorporate birds that are housed together, new bird additions to the aviary or household, recent attendance by the owner to bird shows/fairs, and quarantine procedures.

Once you have the information about the environment and history, there should be a review of the patient's past and current health problems. If the bird was recently purchased, the new owner may not know the entire patient disease history. An investigative phone call to the previous owner may give you or the veterinarian important information that may help make a final diagnosis.

Before an avian patient is restrained to perform a physical exam, an overview of the general disposition is determined from a distance by the technician. The bird should be examined for perching ability, ease of breathing, awareness of the surroundings, and stool characteristics. It is common for birds to have a very liquid stool when excited or in unfamiliar surroundings. The owner should be questioned for any abnormalities in fecal color and consistency. Often a bird is presented in a cage that it commonly stays in and a number of droppings are on the bottom of the cage for the veterinarian or technician to evaluate. If possible, this "hands-off" evaluation is best achieved when looking through a one-way mirror or a small window in the exam room door. The bird will act more natural when it is alone in the room with the owner—rather than with someone it does not trust. Any abnormalities should be noted in the patient's record.

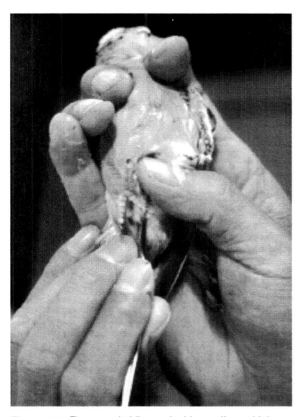

Figure 1-7 The proper holding method for small cage birds.

RESTRAINT

One of the greatest fears for anyone is the capture and restraint of a small bird or a large parrot. The fear when catching a small bird is associated with a sudden unexplained death, while it is the fear of personal injury that most concerns the handler of large parrots. However, it is important to emphasize that it is the rare avian patient that dies from a "heart attack" or fear associated with the capture event. The technician must remember that sick birds are being presented to the veterinary clinic for care and treatment. During the initial assessment and history evaluation, one must decide if the patient is in a condition to be handled for further examination. When an avian patient, or any exotic animal patient, is so ill that capture and restraint may cause death, the owner needs to be fully informed of the possible consequences. To reduce stress on small birds during capture, the overhead light should be turned off after the technician has established the location of the bird. In the dark, birds do not often move or see the hand prior to capture. The lighting of the room should be returned to normal once the patient is in the hands of the technician. This method of capture works extremely well when a bird is free-flying in the room or with large, difficult-to-catch parrots. Small birds (< 120 grams) can be held in one hand. The head is maintained between the forefinger and middle finger as the bird rests in dorsal recumbency in the palm of the hand with the thumb, ring finger, and pinkie loosely holding the body (Figure 1-7).

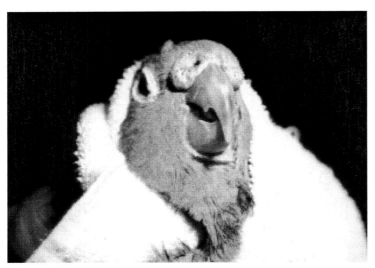

Figure 1-8 Grasping a bird around the neck using an Elizabethan grip.

When working with large parrots, experience and the use of proper capture techniques help to alleviate the fear of having fingers crushed by a large parrot beak. Most injuries occur when the person trying to capture a large parrot is distracted and/or hesitates and is not concentrating on the primary goal of properly restraining the patient. For companion birds, capture should always be achieved through the use of a towel. A towel allows you to hide your hand as it is maneuvered around the back of a bird's neck (Figure 1-8). If the bird has never been captured with a towel or is friendly, the towel should be presented from the front of the animal. The frontal presentation will not scare the bird and allow it to see the towel during capture. The frontal presentation may prevent the bird from developing a future fear of capture. If the bird is difficult to capture, it is recommended to quickly grasp the back of the neck with the toweled hand as the bird is biting the side of the transport carrier. The large bird is held in an Elizabethan grip around the neck, with the thumb and forefinger touching and pressing up against the mandible, the other hand holding the feet, one wing against the body, and the other held by a towel or fingers (Figure 1-9). The Elizabethan grip does not damage the bird's face and gives the handler more control over the beak.

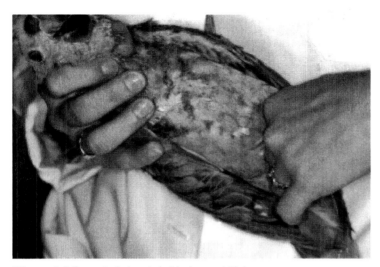

Figure 1-9 Proper technique to hold a large pet bird.

Once a bird is captured with a towel (or in the case of breeder birds, a net or gloves), the patient can be placed in an avian restraint device (Figure 1-10). This Plexiglas® board can restrain birds from the size of a budgerigar to a Hyacinth Macaw. Typically, birds that are placed in the device are less stressed than ones held by veterinary assistants. One area that needs to be addressed when the bird is placed in the restraint board is to prevent the wings from flapping. The veterinary technician should loosely hold the wings against the bird's body to prevent injury to the patient. Birds in the restraint device can be examined and diagnostic samples obtained, including blood and choanal and cloacal cultures.

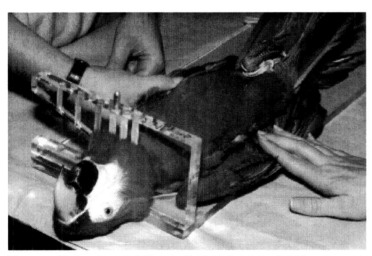

Figure 1-10 An avian restraint board with bird in it. Avian restraint boards adequately restrain birds for physical examinations, diagnostics, sampling, and radiology.

There are many different species of birds that may present to a veterinary clinic. Each species provides different obstacles and dangers to the person trying to capture the patient. If you are not sure how to capture and restrain the animal, please ask someone who knows the technique. This advice will help protect you and the patient from serious injury. Owls, eagles, and hawks have powerful sharp talons that can cause serious puncture wounds. Raptors need to be captured using leather gloves, and feet should be taped prior to an examination. Herons, cranes and egrets have long sharp beaks that are routinely thrust toward the eyes of someone that poses a perceived threat to their well-being. These birds should be captured and restrained by someone who is wearing protective eyewear. Again, if you are not sure how to capture and restrain an avian patient, please ask an experienced technician or veterinarian.

PHYSICAL EXAMINATION

The first and most important information the veterinarian should obtain about the avian patient is the body weight. All exotic animal patients must be weighed on a digital gram scale that measures in 1-gram increments. Tame birds can be placed on a perch that is attached to the base of the scale with Velcro® strips. Untamed birds can be weighed in a container or in the restraint device.

Once the bird has been examined prior to capture and it is determined that the patient is in a condition to be restrained, the veterinarian should perform a "hands-on" physical examination. The feather quality is the first feature that is examined on the bird. Feathers should be examined for abnormal molting, development, damage, abnormal color, ectoparasites, and feather loss. After the feathers, the examiner should start at the head and look straight at the bird, analyzing the beak and eyes for any asymmetry or, in the case of the beak, abnormal wear. The nares are investigated next, primarily searching for any nasal discharge or intranasal growths associated with granulomas.

Ocular examinations are very important, especially on older birds and injured raptor species. The typical ophthalmology assessment includes looking for ocular discharge and eyelid, conjunctival, corneal, anterior chamber, and lens health. The above-mentioned parameters can be examined without using any equipment or a small animal ophthalmoscope. To examine the posterior chamber and retina, a more detailed ocular investigation is required. The more detailed ophthalmology examinations are required for raptors and pet birds that present with head trauma.

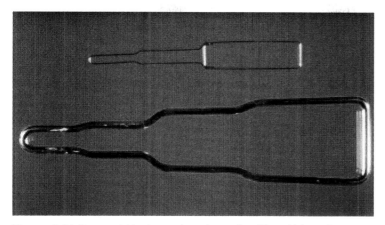

Figure 1-11 Commercial beak speculums for small and large bird species.

Using a beak speculum (Figure 1-11), the oral cavity is observed, including the choanal slit. The terminus of the upper respiratory system, the choanal slit is lined with epithelial projections called papilla. The papilla readily slough in the presence of an upper respiratory infection. Evidence of a chronic upper respiratory infection includes sloughed papilla and a swollen, inflamed choanal slit. The oral cavity should be free of any abscesses, plaques, or necrotic tissue. The glottis is located at the base of the tongue and should also be free of abscesses or epithelial plaques.

Most pet bird species have a dry oral cavity. A dry oral cavity makes it difficult to determine hydration status in these species. Hydration status in avian species should be determined by assessing corneal moisture, globe position in the orbit, skin elasticity through skin tenting, and packed cell volume (PCV).

The crop, or ingluvies, is positioned at the level of the thoracic inlet. Crop stasis, or a large doughy feel to the crop because of undigested food, is often a sign of bacterial ingluvitis. Foreign bodies or trauma associated with hand-feeding may be noted in this area as bruising or a confirmation of a presentation history provided by the owner. If the owner feeds food that is too hot, bruising may occur; or if presentation of the patient is delayed after the thermal burn, necrosis of the crop and skin may be seen. A fistula may form at the location of the thoracic inlet, with the crop adhering to the surface epithelium—causing ingested food to dribble out onto the feathers.

The keel bone is the modified sternum of flighted birds and is the location of the major pectoral muscles. The pectoral muscles on flighted birds can comprise up to 20% of the total body weight. By palpating the pectoral muscles, one can determine the general

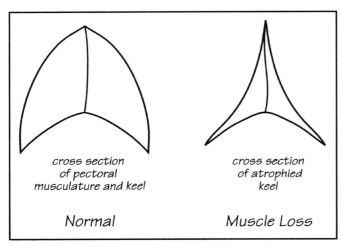

Figure 1-12 Normal keel versus thin keel. Pectoral musculature helps determine the body condition of an avian patient. A full-bodied bird with a well-developed pectoral muscle mass usually indicates good health.

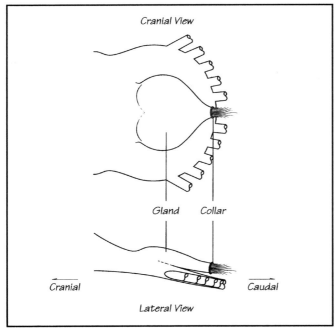

Figure 1-13 The uropygial gland is located at the caudal dorsal aspect of any avian species. This gland aids in feather grooming and waterproofing. It is very well developed in aquatic avian species.

body condition of a companion avian patient. The pectoral muscles should fill the entire space provided by the keel. If the keel is prominent, the bird is considered underweight (Figure 1-12).

In the caudal areas of a bird's body, very few diagnostic observations can be made because of the large surface area of the keel bone. Palpation of the caudal coelomic cavity behind the keel bone may reveal hepatomegly associated with a tumor, an egg in the reproductive tract, or ascites resulting from internal ovulation. Cranial to the insertion of the tail feathers on the dorsal midline is the location of the uropygial or preen gland (Figure 1-13). The uropygial gland is absent in some companion avian species, e.g., the Amazon Parrot, but well-developed in waterfowl. The gland is typically a bilobed structure with a papilla emanating from the center that may include a tuft of feathers. Any bleeding, inflammation, or asymmetry to this gland is abnormal.

Most birds project their waste from the body; therefore, the feathers around the vent are normally clean. Any soiling or pasting of waste noted around the vent should be noted as abnormal. The vent and cloaca should be examined for papillomas (cloacal warts), especially in larger parrots and macaws. A cotton-tipped applicator can be placed in the cloaca, carefully everting the structure to observe the mucocutaneous junction. The normal appearance should be smooth, but if any roughness is observed on the tissue surface, further testing is required. By using 5% acetic acid (vinegar) applied to a cotton-tipped applicator and placing the solution on the questionable surface, one can obtain a tentative diagnosis. If the mucous surface of the cloaca is intact, the vinegar will not adhere, but if the surface is compromised by papillomas, the surface will turn white.

The wings and legs are the last body structures to be examined after the bird is osculated. Bird's lungs are located on the ventral aspect of the thoracic vertebra. By locating the head of the stethoscope on the dorsal body wall in this area, one may listen for any abnormal respiratory sounds. The heart is best osculated on the left lateral body wall under the wing in the axillary region. Osculated heart murmurs in companion avian species, especially cockatoos, have been diagnosed with ventricular septal defects. The wings and legs are examined for fractures, joint integrity, and range of motion. The nails and plantar surface of the feet are the final areas that are assessed for any abnormal physical characteristics.

As with other animals, after the examination is complete, any abnormal findings are recorded and a list of differential diagnoses is established. Based on the top differential diagnoses, diagnostic tests are prioritized to confirm a diagnosis or to determine the severity of disease.

"PUT IT DOWN"

If the bird has an increased respiratory rate, excessive vocalization and/or has difficulty breathing during the physical examination, the bird may have to be "put down" until it is able to withstand the rigors of the evaluation process.

Criteria used to back off evaluating an avian patient until a later time:[1]

- If the bird is panting or breathing rapidly, first alter the grip on the head, so the head is free to move. The bird should immediately begin to turn its head in search of something to bite. If it does not, PUT IT DOWN.

- A paper towel, or a corner of the towel being used to restrain the bird, can be placed into its mouth. It should immediately begin to bite at this, demonstrating that it has sufficient oxygen reserves to do so. If it lets the material lay lamely in its mouth, PUT IT DOWN.

- Have the bird grasp your hand or finger with both of its feet. (This should be part of the physical examination, to determine symmetry and strength of grip). If the bird's grip is weak, or nonexistent, PUT IT DOWN.

- If the bird's eyes close during the physical examination PUT IT DOWN. Conversely, do not be reassured if the bird has its eyes open—many birds have held their eyes open as they drew their last breath.

- If in doubt—PUT IT DOWN. Return the bird to the location (cage, owner) where it is most comfortable, and observe it while discussing possible etiologies for the bird's decreased respiratory capacity with the owner.

DIAGNOSTIC SAMPLING

BLOOD COLLECTION

Many veterinarians and veterinary technicians think that it is close to impossible to obtain any usable quantity of blood from an avian patient without compromising its health or killing the bird. This is a totally false assumption that has been perpetuated within the profession. With the technology available today, blood samples can be easily obtained (even from the smallest avian patient) that will provide usable diagnostic information. Approximately 1% of the bird's blood volume can be taken safely for diagnostic testing, or 1 ml/100 grams body weight.

Each particular avian species has a vein that is recommended as the choice site for blood collection. In companion avian species, the vein of choice for blood collection is the right jugular vein. Birds do have a left jugular vein, but it is less developed than the right side. Other veins or venous sinuses that can be used for blood collection in avian patients include the basilic vein, median metatarsal vein, or the occipital venous

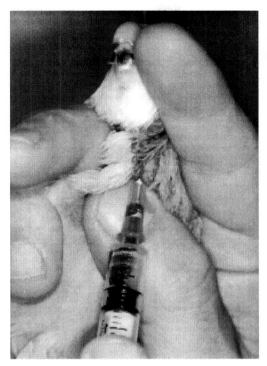

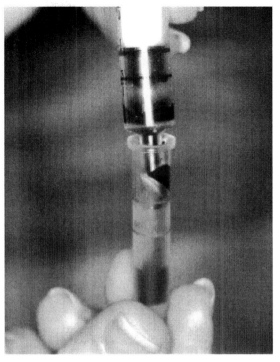

Figure 1-14 One-handed blood draw. Proper technique is being used in drawing blood from the right jugular vein.

Figure 1-15 Microtainer® tubes. This is a typical 0.5ml blood collection tube used in avian diagnostic testing.

sinus. Blood collection techniques used for other animals should be followed with avian patients. The right jugular vein can be observed in a featherless tract of epithelium in the right lateral cervical region. A 3-cc syringe with a 26-gauge needle is recommended as the instrument of choice for birds weighing more than 30 grams and less than 2 kilograms. For birds less than 30 grams, a 1-cc syringe is recommended, because of the low volume of blood that can be safely removed from the patient (Figure 1-14). Unless the patient is extremely fractious, no general anesthesia is required when drawing blood. Once the blood has been retrieved in the syringe, it should be placed in a Microtainer® tube (Becton Dickinson Microbiology Systems, Cockeysville, MD) and gently agitated to allow exposure to the anticoagulant (Figure 1-15). The agitation of the blood in the collection tube should take place quickly because avian blood has a tendency to rapidly coagulate. Table 1-1 lists the hematologic reference ranges for parrot species, and Table 1-2 lists the plasma biochemical reference ranges for common parrot species. For hematologic testing, or complete blood counts (CBC), a purple top Microtainer® tube is recommended (Table 1-1), and for plasma biochemistries, a green top Microtainer® tube should be used (Table 1-2).[2]

Table 1-1
Avian Hematologic Reference Ranges[2]

Value	African Grey Parrot	Amazon Parrot	Budgerigar	Cockatiel	Cockatoo	Conure	Eclectus Parrot	Lovebird	Macaw	Pionus	Quaker Parrot
Hematocrit (%)	42 - 53	43 - 49	44 - 54	43 - 58	42 - 51	43 - 56	43 - 50	43 - 55	43 - 54	43 - 54	- - - -
Red blood cells (x10^6/ml)	2.80 - 3.36	2.33 - 2.95	3.90 - 4.70	3.8 - 4.58	2.50 - 2.95	3.13 - 3.94	2.7 - 3.1	2.63 - 3.50	- - - -	2.7 - 3.5	- - - -
Hemoglobin (g/dl)	15.1 - 16.9	14.4 - 16.7	13.4 - 15.3	12.1 - 14.6	12.0 - 14.8	12.1 - 14.8	14.1 - 16.0	11.9 - 15.1	- - - -	14.2 - 15.5	- - - -
Mean corpuscular volume (fl)	143 - 155	163 - 170	115 - 124	128 - 142	154 - 170	135 - 147	157 - 170	155 - 166	- - - -	154 - 164	- - - -
Mean corpuscular hemoglobin (g/dl)	32.3 - 45.6	49.8 - 58.2	25.9 - 30.9	24.9 - 36.0	45.0 - 55.5	30.0 - 40.1	51.3 - 54.2	40 - 48	- - - -	41.4 - 46.0	- - - -
Mean corp. Hb concentration (g/dl)	23.16 - 31.78	32.8 - 35.31	19.80 - 26.75	18.91 - 25.61	24.12 - 32.91	23.5 - 28.6	31.2 - 34.0	21.9 - 29.3	- - - -	25.8 - 28.7	- - - -
White blood cells (x10^3/ml)	6.0 - 13.0	5.0 - 12.5	3.0 - 8.0	5.0 - 9.0	5.0 - 12.0	4.0 - 9.0	9.0 - 15.0	3.0 - 8.0	7.0 - 12.0	5.0 - 13.0	8.0 - 17.0
Heterophils (%)	45 - 72	32 - 71	41 - 67	47 - 72	45 - 72	45 - 72	46 - 70	41 - 71	48 - 72	55 - 74	47 - 70
Lymphocytes (%)	25 - 50	20 - 65	22 - 58	27 - 58	20 - 50	22 - 49	23 - 57	28 - 52	18 - 52	19 - 70	20 - 63
Monocytes (%)	0 - 1	0 - 1	0 - 2	0 - 1	0 - 1	0 - 1	0 - 1	0 - 1	0 - 1	0 - 1	0 - 4
Basophils (%)	0 - 1	0 - 2	0 - 2	0 - 1	0 - 1	0 - 2	0 - 1	0 - 1	0 - 1	0 - 1	0 - 3
Eosinophils (%)	0 - 1	0 - 0.05	0 - 0.05	0 - 2	0 - 2	0 - 1	0 - 1	0 - 1	0 - 1	0 - 1	0 - 4

Table 1-2
Avian Plasma Biochemical Reference Ranges [2]

Values	African Grey Parrot	Amazon Parrot	Budgerigar	Cockatiel	Cockatoo	Conure	Eclectus Parrot	Lovebird	Macaw
Albumin (g/dl)	0.2 - 2.4	0.3 - 2.4	0.9 - 1.2	0.8 - 1.8	0.3 - 0.9	0.3 - 0.9	1.1 - 2	0.3 - 0.9	0.3 - 2.4
Alkaline phosphate (U/L)	12 - 92	8 - 100	24 - 96	12 - 100	24 - 104	24 - 104	32 - 111	- - - -	12 - 100
Amylase (U/L)	415 - 626	184 - 478	302 - 560	113 - 870	288 - 876	192 - 954	562 - 684	- - - -	239 - 564
Aspartate aminotransferase [AST] (U/L)	112 - 339	155 - 380	160 - 372	130 - 390	145 - 346	147 - 360	144 - 339	130 - 343	60 - 165
Bile acids (mol/L)	12 - 85	35 - 144	35 - 110	45 - 105	37 - 98	35 - 90	30 - 110	34 - 88	30 - 80
Calcium (mg/dl)	8.3 - 11.7	8.5 - 13.0	8.5 - 11.0	8.3 - 10.9	8.4 - 11.0	8.4 - 11.0	8.1 - 11.9	8.6 - 11.5	8.3 - 11.0
Cholesterol (mg/dl)	100 - 250	150 - 220	120 - 220	90 - 195	90 - 200	83 - 190	100 - 261	125 - 195	96 - 264
Creatine kinase [CK] (U/L)	120 - 410	120 - 410	120 - 360	167 - 420	150 - 400	140 - 397	132 - 410	160 - 320	90 - 360
Creatinine (mg/dl)	0.1 - 0.5	- - - -	- - - -	0.1 - 0.5	0.1 - 0.8	0.1 - 0.8	- - - -	0.1 - 0.8	0.1 - 0.7
Globulin (g/dl)	1.2 - 3.6	1.6 - 3.7	1.1 - 1.7	2.5 - 3.8	2.5 - 3.8	2.5 - 3.8	2 - 3.32	2.5 - 3.8	2.1 - 3.8
Glucose (mg/dl)	280 - 354	250 - 370	210 - 450	230 - 440	210 - 410	230 - 400	- - - -	210 - 390	210 - 360
Phosphorus (mg/dl)	3.5 - 6.9	- - - -	3.7 - 7.1	4.0 - 7.7	4.2 - 7.8	4.0 - 7.9	- - - -	- - - -	4.0 - 7.8
Protein, plasma (g/dl)	2.7 - 4.4	2.6 - 4.5	2.1 - 4.3	2.1 - 4.8	2.6 - 2.8	2.4 - 4.9	3.2 - 4.3	1.8 - 3.7	2.4 - 4.4
Uric acid (mg/dl)	1.9 - 9.7	2.3 - 9.8	4.0 - 12.2	3.5 - 10.4	3.6 - 10.7	2.7 - 10.2	2.0 - 11.0	3.2 - 10.2	1.5 - 11.0

BONE MARROW ASPIRATION

The site of choice in avian patients for bone marrow aspiration is the proximal tibiotarsal bone. A 22-gauge 1.5" spinal needle is placed at the lateral aspect of the proximal tibiotarsal bone of an anesthetized patient (Figure 1-16). The needle is slowly rotated with gentle pressure toward the medullary cavity. When a sudden reduction of pressure is felt, the medullary cavity has been reached, and the technician then removes the stylet of the spinal needle. A 6-cc syringe is placed on the needle and bone marrow is drawn into the needle with short quick pulls on the plunger. Pressure is released off the plunger, and the needle removed from the bone. Remove the needle from the syringe and draw about 4–5-cc of air into the syringe, place the needle back on the syringe, and eject needle contents on a clean microscope slide.

MICROBIOLOGY

Microbiological sampling techniques that are used on other animals can be applied to the avian patient. Regular and mini-tipped culturettes are used, depending on the size of the orifice being sampled. It is recommended that the larger culturette be used whenever possible to increase the chances of isolating a pathogenic organism. Common sites cultured in avian patients include the choana, crop, and cloaca (terminus of the digestive tract). Cultures can also be taken of internal lesions through an endoscopic cannula or biopsy samples of abnormal tissue.

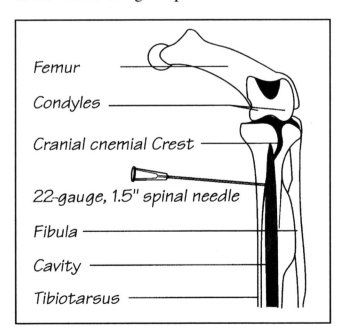

Femur

Condyles

Cranial cnemial Crest

22-gauge, 1.5" spinal needle

Fibula

Cavity

Tibiotarsus

Figure 1-16 Proximal tibiotarsal bone. This is the site of choice for bone marrow aspiration.

Most of the organisms associated with avian disease are aerobic, and this is the most common diagnostic growth test. If there is a possibility of an anaerobic organism causing disease in the patient, the laboratory should be made aware of the differential diagnosis to properly prepare the sample for isolation of that class of bacteria. The same protocol should be followed for fungal and mycobacterium isolation and identification.

Common pathogenic bacterial isolates in companion avian species include, some *E. coli* and *Enterobacter* spp., *Pseudomonas* spp., *Klebsiella* spp., and in some cases, *Mycobacterium avium. Aspergillus* spp. is often found in raptors and waterfowl that are stressed through rehabilitation or oil spill clean-up procedures. Common fungal infections in companion avian species also include *Aspergillus* spp. and *Candida albicans*. The first diagnostic test that may be performed is a Gram's stain on the fecal material. The Gram's staining of fecal material or crop contents will help the veterinarian assess gastrointestinal health through determination of current flora within the digestive system. Companion avian species should have a majority of Gram-positive rods and very few, if any, *Candida albicans* organisms. If any Gram-negative rods are noted on the stain, a total evaluation of the patient should be made to determine the significance of the finding. A patient with diarrhea or that is anorexic upon presentation may be affected by the abnormal percentage of Gram-negative organisms and further testing should be initiated. Birds showing no abnormal signs usually are not affected by an abnormal bacterial population, but should be monitored and/or tested to establish baseline data.

RADIOLOGY

Companion avian species, in most cases, should be radiographed under general anesthesia on an avian restraint board. By radiographing an avian patient under general anesthesia, using isoflurane or sevoflurane, the ability to obtain quality radiographs with minimal stress to the bird is greatly increased. Proper assessment of the patient is required to determine the ability of the animal to withstand this procedure. Common presentations that require radiographs include trauma, fractures, heavy metal toxicosis, respiratory distress, gastrointestinal stasis (proventricular dilatation disease), swallowing a foreign body, and nonspecific neurologic signs. High-detail film is a must when radiographing any small exotic animal species, especially birds. The same radiology techniques used for other companion animals need to be followed with avian species. This would include always getting two views, on perpendicular planes, of the desired area of interest.

PARASITOLOGY

Ectoparasites

As discussed earlier, many new bird owners believe that all avian species commonly have external parasites, particularly lice. It is important that the veterinary clinic personnel inform these owners that it is rare for pet avian species to become infested with any type of external parasite. Caged birds are seldom exposed to environments where they would contact the parasites that live on the skin or feathers. Outdoor aviaries, where people breed parrot species, might provide the opportunity for the transmission of lice or mites from infested native birds. Raptors, waterfowl, and other fowl will commonly present with ectoparasites at which time the owner should initiate treatment of the bird and environment. Most of the external parasites that are mentioned in this section can be treated with ivermectin (Ivomec, Merck AgVet Division, Rahway, NJ, 0.2 mg/kg, orally or subcutaneously for 2 to 3 treatments, 14 days apart).

If birds are maintained indoors, there is very little chance of exposure to external parasites. Aviary birds and other avian species that are maintained in flights have a better chance of being diagnosed with parasitic arthropods. There are two common ectoparasites that infest caged birds: *Sternostoma tracheacolum* and *Knemidokoptes* spp. *Sternostoma tracheacolum* is also known as the tracheal/air sac mite, and it mainly affects canaries and finches. The birds diagnosed with the tracheal mite show signs of respiratory distress and have an audible clicking sound when breathing. Ivermectin is the treatment of choice for birds infested with *Sternostoma tracheacolum*.

Knemidokoptes spp. lives in the featherless areas around the face and legs (Figure 1-17). Common names for these arthropod parasites are scaly face and/or scaly leg mites. The names are derived from the irritation of the surface epithelium that causes a hyperkeratosis of the affected skin and beak. Budgerigars are the most common pet birds to be diagnosed with *Knemidokoptes* spp., although other species may be susceptible, particularly eclectus parrots and canaries. As with tracheal mites, ivermectin is the treatment of choice for *Knemidokoptes* spp.

Chewing lice of the order *Mallophaga* and domestic poultry mites *Dermanyssus gallinae* and *Ornithodoros sylviarum* may affect parrot species that live outdoors in breeding flights. Environmental cleaning is very important in trying to prevent reinfestation of the lice and mites. A 5% carbaryl powder may be used in conjunction with ivermectin therapy to treat infested birds.

Internal Parasites

As with external parasites, internal parasites are uncommon in companion birds that are hand-raised and maintained indoors. Birds that live in breeding flights, and especially birds that have access to the ground, have a better chance for exposure to internal parasite eggs and larvae. All birds should have direct fecal and fecal flotation examinations as part of a complete health check. Psittacine species infected with the protozoan parasite *Giardia psittaci* will present with chronic to intermittent watery diarrhea and with loose, malodorous mucoid stools.[3] Another protozoan parasite that is diagnosed in avian patients (particularly doves, pigeons, and raptors) is *Trichomonas gallinae*. Whereas giardiasis is associated with the intestinal tract, trichomoniasis is found as white plaques or necrotic masses in the mouth and esophagus.[1] Metronidazole (Flagyl, G. D. Searle Co., Chicago, IL) can be used to treat both *Giardia psittaci* and *Trichomonas gallinae*.

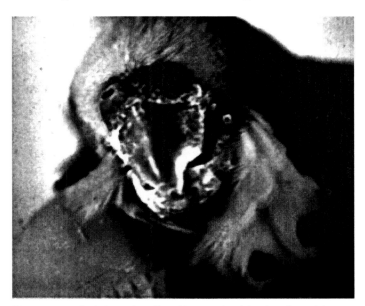

Figure 1-17 Scaly face mites. The white areas involving the edges of the upper beak and lower beak are consistent with hyperkeritosis. This condition is attributed to scaly face mite infestation and is commonly seen in budgerigars.

Two coccidian parasites may be diagnosed in caged birds. *Atoxoplasma* spp. organisms are diagnosed in canaries, finches, and mynah birds. The diagnosis is usually made during a pathology examination of a dead juvenile bird that dies shortly after appearing depressed and fluffed. *Atoxoplasma* spp. organisms are shed in the feces of adults that show no signs of infection. Treatment of any coccidian disease is difficult; often the best outcome is a reduction of shedding and exposure to unaffected birds. Trimethoprim/ sulfadiazine (Roche Pharmaceuticals, Nutley, NJ) is the recommended treatment for avian coccidian parasitic diseases. *Sarcocystis falcatula* is the other coccidian parasite diagnosed in companion avian species. This parasite usually affects aviary birds housed outdoors in breeding flights. The life cycle of *Sarcocystis falcatula* involves the opossum (*Didelphis virginiana*) and cockroaches. As with *Atoxoplasma* spp., *Sarcocystis falcatula* is usually diagnosed during a pathology examination on a dead bird. The extensive life cycle requirements of the parasite make environmental management extremely important if the owner wants to prevent exposure and infection within an aviary.

Hemoproteus spp., *Plasmodium* spp., and *Leukocytozoon* spp. are parasites that may be noted in red blood cells of wild-caught psittacine species, raptors, doves, and pigeons. These parasites are transmitted through the bite of infected arthropods. Unless there is an overwhelming infestation of these parasites, treatment is not recommended.

Before the Wild Bird Conservation Act was passed in the early 1990s, a vast number of large psittacine species were being imported into the United States. Wild-caught cockatoo species and African Grey Parrots were often diagnosed with tapeworms. With the passage of the conservation act, the number of these species being diagnosed with cestodes has diminished. Treatment of cestode infestations can be accomplished with praziquantel (Droncit, Haver/Diamond Scientific, Shawnee, KS).

Nematodes, as with most of the parasites that affect avian species, commonly affect birds that live in outdoor environments. Ascarids have a direct life cycle, in which simply ingesting eggs can infect a bird, while *Capillaria* spp. and *Syngamus trachea* need earthworms as an intermediate host. Ascarids and *Capillaria* spp. live in the intestinal tract, and *Syngamus trachea* are found in the oral cavity and esophagus. Birds infested with intestinal parasites will be depressed and emaciated. In most cases, nematode eggs are shed in the feces and can be seen in a fecal flotation exam. It is important to treat the bird and, if possible, the environment.

SURGICAL AND ANESTHETIC ASSISTANCE

Surgical preparation techniques are similar for birds as for other species treated at a small animal hospital. There are a few main differences regarding avian species, and they will be covered in this section. The normal body temperature for birds ranges between 103–105°F. To maintain this high body temperature, birds eat often and the food rapidly passes through the digestive tract. For this reason, fasting is only recommended for two hours prior to surgery. Using isoflurane or sevoflurane anesthesia, birds are induced via a facemask and then intubated with a noncuffed endotracheal tube. A noncuffed endotracheal tube is recommended because most avian species have complete tracheal rings and an inflated cuff may induce pressure necrosis on the epithelium lining of the trachea. The glottis is readily observed at the base of the tongue once this anatomical structure is extended using hemostats. The neck should be extended when placing the endotracheal tube into the recommended position, about the mid-cervical region. It must be remembered that the syrinx, or voice box, of avian species is located at the tracheal bifurcation. With the syrinx located at this level in the respiratory tract, a patient may still vocalize—even with proper placement of the endotracheal tube. If head surgery needs to be performed or if there is a blockage of the trachea, an air sac cannulation can take place to provide oxygen or anesthesia into the respiratory system. Isoflurane anesthesia has a side effect of respiratory depression; therefore, bagging the patient 2 to 3 times a minute will help offset any problems caused by the anesthetic gas.

The surgical plane of anesthesia and patient status can be monitored by the palpebral and pedal reflexes, heart and respiration rate, and by plucking feathers. To prepare a surgical site on the body, feathers must be plucked in the direction opposite of the way they lay (against the grain). A wide area must be plucked and feathers removed from the surgical field with a handheld vacuum device. Feathers have the amazing tendency to reappear in the surgical field if not properly removed. Once feathers are removed from the surgical site, the skin is well exposed for the procedure. Site preparation is much less involved in birds than mammalian species that have been clipped. A surgical scrub should involve two scrubs using a commercial surgical scrub product and sterile saline. Often radiosurgical or electrocautery units are used in avian surgical procedures. If alcohol is part of the scrub procedure, the bird will be in flames when the surgeon initiates the incision. Alcohol also contributes to hypothermia in the patient, increasing surgical complications for the anesthetist. To monitor body temperature, an esophageal thermometer works much better than a cloacal probe. To maintain heat, a water blanket is placed under the patient and a heat lamp over the patient—out of the surgeon's field of view. Clear plastic drapes help the anesthetist monitor the patient during surgery. The plastic drapes help in observing the bird's respiration, but may contribute to hyperthermia. Any change in the patient's temperature is best monitored with a thermometer, and actions should be quickly taken to stabilize the body temperature into the normal range. A respiratory monitor that is attached to the tracheal tube and the tube extending from the anesthesia machine will give audible sounds with each breath. These monitors can be used on birds that are as small as budgerigars to birds that are as large as an ostrich. The respiratory monitor will help the anesthetist determine if the bird is going into a deeper plane of anesthesia or is becoming "light."

Birds should recover quickly from gas anesthesia. Once the vaporizer is turned off, oxygen should be administered until the patient shows signs of recovery. During recovery, the bird must be maintained in an incubator unit to help with body temperature stabilization.

HEALTH MAINTENANCE AND DISEASES

This section will review the common avian diseases seen in veterinary practice. An overview of etiology, treatment, and prevention will follow a brief description of the disease presentation.

RESPIRATORY AND GASTROINTESTINAL BACTERIAL/FUNGAL INFECTIONS

Birds have a well-developed respiratory system that is composed of 4 paired and 1 unpaired air sac(s) and an extensive upper respiratory sinus (infraorbital). Most people assume that the only diet a bird should eat is seed. As a result, many pet birds are fed a vitamin deficient diet, especially in vitamin A. Since vitamin A is an integral component of epithelial health, a companion bird that is suffering from hypovitaminosis A will have a compromised respiratory and gastrointestinal epithelium. The compromised epithelial surface provides an environment for microorganisms to adhere and infect the bird. External stress factors affect the immune system of birds, which reduces their internal ability to fight the infection or aid antibiotic treatment. Birds that are immature, old, being transported, quarantined, or in shows are the most susceptible to bacteria and fungal infections. Some avian species are able to handle external stresses better than others. The Gyrfalcon and Red-tailed Hawk commonly become infected with *Aspergillus* spp. infections, while other raptors are less susceptible to this often-fatal fungal infection.

To treat bacterial and fungal infections it is essential to identify the organism and find out what drug(s) will effectively treat the disease. Stabilization of the patient and boosting its physiologic status through supportive care will aid in the successful treatment of these cases. If birds are not diagnosed or treated properly for the appropriate length of time, the bacterial and fungal infections can kill the patient or cause irreversible anatomic damage.

FEATHER PICKING AND FEATHER LOSS

One of the most frustrating avian case presentations for veterinarians to treat is a bird suffering from feather loss or self-inflicted feather picking. If the head feathers are intact, this usually means that the animal is pulling or traumatizing its own feathers. If the head feathers are also affected, this often indicates a generalized health problem. It is the responsibility of the veterinarian to give the bird with feather loss a complete physical examination, incorporating a good owner history, to make sure there are no treatable medical problems before making a diagnosis of psychological feather picking.

A number of parasitic, infectious, and noninfectious diseases may initiate and perpetuate feather loss in a pet bird. It is only through the thorough and diligent understanding of a case that the correct treatment is provided to the patient. If it is determined that the problem is psychological, environmental and nutritional changes can be recommended to the owner for a possible resolution of the problem. If the initial recommendations are unsuccessful, veterinarians may prescribe psychotropic, antidepressant, and antihistamine drugs. Currently, researchers are investigating the possibility of hypersensitivity reactions in pet birds and agents that may cause allergic reactions. Elizabethan collars have been used with some success in preventing birds from pulling feathers. Elizabethan collars are just a physical barrier for the birds and do not actually treat the underlying cause of feather picking; therefore, the primary cause should be identified and treated for long-lasting resolution of this frustrating disease.

TRAUMA

There are many situations in which birds can become injured through traumatic accidents. Flying into ceiling fans, sliding glass doors, walls and cars, getting burned in water or being burned by hand-feeding formula, or being bitten by a cagemate (or other animal such as a dog or cat) are the most common causes of traumatic injury to avian patients. Upon presentation, the patient should be quickly assessed and stabilized. Only when the patient is stabilized should extensive treatment or diagnostics take place. Maintaining hydration status and treating shock, parasites, and infection are required for serious injuries. Educating owners about common household hazards and trimming a bird's wings will reduce the incidents of traumatic injury.

EGG-BINDING

Dystocia, or egg-binding, is the inability of a hen to complete the process of laying an egg. The egg usually is caught in the shell-gland of the oviduct and needs to be removed by the veterinarian. Cockatiels are one of the most common pet bird species that present with this problem. Treatment for egg-binding includes heat, humidity, calcium, oxytocin, and propulcid. After the hen has been stabilized and the therapeutic agents have been given an appropriate length of time to take effect, a slow, gentle push on the egg toward the cloaca often aids in its expulsion from the vent. In birds that have a history of egg-binding or laying a large number of eggs, a salpingoectomy is advised to prevent a possible life-threatening condition in the future.

HEAVY METAL TOXICOSIS

Lead and zinc are the most common heavy metal toxicities that affect pet birds. Companion birds come into contact with lead from peeling paint, weights, toys, solder, wine caps, and lead headed nails. Zinc exposure is usually through galvanized wire and containers and toys. If a bird presents with neurologic signs, a heavy metal screen should be submitted. Zinc toxicity is more nonspecific, usually presenting as gastroenteritis. Radiographs often identify heavy metal foreign bodies within the gastrointestinal tract. Chelation therapy may be initiated immediately if heavy metal toxicosis is suspected. The use of calcium disodium ethylenediaminetetracetate (CaEDTA) should be carefully monitored, since it has been reported to cause gastrointestinal and renal toxicosis.[4] Removal of the foreign body(s) through the use of laxatives or surgery will accelerate the treatment process. Uptake of the serologic heavy metal by bone tissue will often cause a relapse of the disease after the initial treatment, because the body will absorb the dead bone cells containing the material when they die. The relapse condition must be mentioned to the owner—noting that periodic rechecks and blood testing will monitor the patient's condition until the danger is over, which is often more than a six-month period.

GROOMING

Bird owners are constantly seeking quality health care for their birds. This health care includes professional grooming services. For many veterinary practices, this is understood for dogs and to a lesser extent cats, but not avian species. One of the most common companion bird presentations to veterinary clinics is for grooming services. Grooming for birds includes beak, feather, and nail trims.

Parrots have a natural overbite, which may be considered overgrowth by the owner. The clinic should have a book or reference guide that shows normal birds, giving the groomer an idea of proper beak length. Malocclusion of the beak from trauma, parasites, or developmental abnormalities will cause the beak to grow off center, predisposing the structure to become overgrown. Using a motor driven hobby tool, the beak can be shaped back into a normal appearance (Figure 1-18). The final result of the beak trim will depend on the anatomy one has to work with, based on the patient's history. Normally, the beak will grow from the underlying germinal epithelium covering the bone that provides the beak its foundation. As the beak epithelium grows out, it may do so in an irregular pattern, which is normal, but may not give the surface a smooth character that is desir-

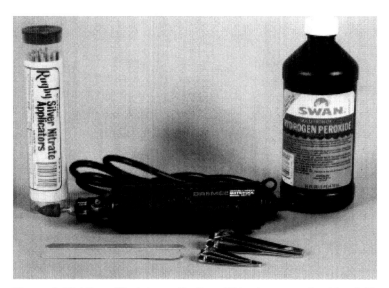

Figure 1-18 A Dremel® tool shown with other nail trimming accessories. A handheld, motor-driven tool is commonly used to groom beaks and trim toenails of larger pet birds.

able to the owner. Carefully applying the stone bit of the motor tool over the irregular areas will smooth out the beak. If the groomer puts too much pressure on the beak, the underlying vascular layer will be compromised and bleeding will occur. To smooth the lower beak, place the tip of the upper beak into the lower beak. Practice and experience will help to improve beak-grooming techniques, especially on larger parrots and macaws. An application of mineral oil will shine and moisten the beak surface and provide a nice presentation for the owner.

Owners may have many reasons for wanting their bird's wing feathers trimmed. The main reason is to restrict flight capabilities, thereby preventing an unwanted escape. Often, birds that are flighted will be more independent, spending less quality time with the owner, and increasing the possibility of flying into walls, ceiling fans, and glass doors. The owner should always be cautioned that trimming a bird's wing feathers will restrict flight, but will not prevent it. Precautions against flight should always be maintained when the bird is outdoors. In recent years,

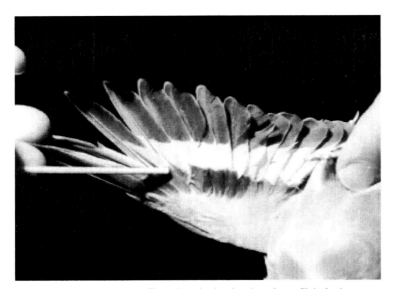

Figure 1-19 Flight feathers. The pointer is showing the primary flight feathers, which are commonly trimmed to restrict the pet bird's flight.

body harnesses have been made for pet birds, and these should be placed on a bird at an early age to expedite recognition and acceptance of these devices. The groomer should ask how the owner would like the wing feathers trimmed and what he wants to accomplish with the restricted flight. The more restrictions an owner places on a nonflighted bird, the greater the number of feathers that will need to be trimmed. The main feathers trimmed are the primary flights on both wings and, to a lesser extent, the secondary flight feathers (Figure 1-19). The feathers should be trimmed under the dorsal covert feathers so the cut feather cannot be seen when the wing is in the normal position. Adequate flight restriction can be obtained in short, fat birds (e.g., Amazon

Parrots, African Grey Parrots) with bilateral trimming of the primary flight feathers. In young African Grey Parrots, this is extremely important because they often fall and cut open their chest over the keel bone. Many Amazon Parrots have pretty orange secondary flight feathers that owners like to keep. Long, thin birds (e.g., cockatiels and conures) need to have the primary and secondary flight feathers trimmed to achieve an adequate flight restriction. Many companion avian species need their wings trimmed twice a year.

Blood feathers are new growing feathers ensheathed and engorged with blood that is carrying nutrient to the developing structure (Figure 1-20). If a primary or secondary blood feather is cut or broken, grasp the base of the feather with hemostats and pull straight out. Digital pressure should be applied to the feather follicle for 2 to 3 minutes to aid in hemostasis.

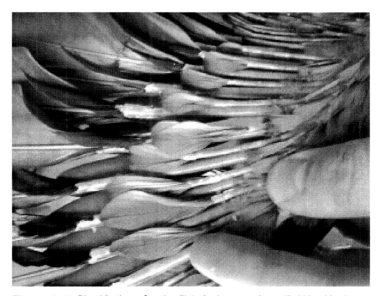

Figure 1-20 Blood feathers. Growing flight feathers are often called blood feathers because the ensheathed, developing feather is nourished by a significant blood supply.

Nail trimming is usually an owner request, and not necessarily needed to provide good health maintenance. Bird nails can become very sharp, enabling a bird to hold on to the perch. Some birds, such as Cockatoo species, have quick-growing nails that curl around, becoming entangled in the cage bars. The nails should be bluntly trimmed to the level of the plantar surface of the foot with a motor-driven hobby tool. If bleeding continues after the trim, silver nitrate tipped wooden applicator sticks are recommended for hemostasis. Young birds' nails have a tendency to bleed more often than older birds'. The nails should be trimmed when the bird is hurting the owner or when there is excessive overgrowth.

BIRD BANDS AND MICROCHIPPING

Companion birds are required to be identified, as stated by the Wild Bird Conservation Act. The most common method of identifying pet and cage birds is by leg bands. Unfortunately, leg bands often become entangled in cage structures and toys. We recommend removing the band and inserting a microchip into the pectoral muscle. By inserting a microchip, leg injury or possible death is averted, and the bird is identified.

OTHER DISEASES

There are many other diseases that infect companion avian species. Common viral diseases include polyoma virus, psittacine beak, and feather disease. Although not identified at this time as a virus, papallomatosis is also diagnosed in large parrot species and macaws. There are tests available to identify polyoma virus, psittacine beak, and feather disease; it is recommended to use a reputable diagnostic laboratory and to provide this service to your clients. A vaccine for polyoma virus is available to protect birds from this devastating disease (Biomune, Lenexa, KS). Vaccinate young birds and older birds to maintain aviary health and the reputation of bird breeders.

ZOONOTIC DISEASES

The primary zoonotic disease associated with pet birds is *Chlamydia psittaci*. Avian chlamydiosis is an intracellular bacterium that presents as a number of disease conditions in birds, but is a respiratory condition in humans. The organism is spread through respiratory secretions and fecal material from infected birds. If an owner develops spiking temperature episodes and a chronic respiratory condition, a physician must be notified of the ownership of birds. There is a publication from the Centers for Disease Control and Prevention that outlines human and avian disease conditions, diagnostic methods, and treatment regimes.[5]

REFERENCES

1.   Lightfoot, T. "Avoiding Disaster in the Critical Patient." Proceedings of the Annual Conference, Association. of Avian Veterinarians, 1998: 265–271.
2.   Altman, R.B., Clubb, S.L., and Dorrestein, G.M. "Hematologic and Plasma Biochemical Reference Ranges of Common Psittacine Species." In Quesenberry, K.E., eds. *Avian Medicine and Surgery*. Philadelphia: W.B. Saunders, 1997: 1005–7.

3. Clyde, V.L. and Patton, S. "Diagnosis, Treatment, and Control of Common Parasites in Companion and Aviary Birds." Seminar in Avian and Exotic Pet Medicine 5, (2) (1996): 52–64.

4. McDonald, S.E. "Lead Poisoning in Psittacine Birds." In Kirk, R.W., ed. *Current Veterinary Therapy IX, Small Animal Practice*, Philadelphia: WB Saunders, 1988: 713–718.

5. Centers for Disease Control and Prevention. "Compendium of Measures to Control *Chlamydia psittaci* Infection Among Humans (Psittacosis) and Pet Birds (Avian chlamydiosis), 1998." (No. RR-10), *Morbidity and Mortality Weekly Report,* 1998: 47.

CHAPTER 2

REPTILES AND AMPHIBIANS

INTRODUCTION

Reptiles and amphibians continue to gain in popularity in the pet trade. A national pet survey estimated that there are 7.5 million homes reporting ownership of at least one reptile. The increased number of animals being maintained in captivity has expanded the need for qualified veterinarians and veterinary technicians to provide the quality medical and surgical care that pet owners have come to expect from our profession. A certified veterinary technician with experience in working with these animals will prove to be valuable in the employment market.

TAXONOMY

Proper identification of a reptile or amphibian is essential to case management. As a veterinary technician, you may be expected to provide your client with information about the natural history of an animal and to make suggestions regarding the environmental and nutritional needs of that particular animal. Unfortunately, many reptiles have been assigned 3–4 different common names depending on who collected or sold a particular animal. It is not uncommon to enter different pet stores and find the same species being sold under different names. Clients may become frustrated while researching the particular needs of an animal if they are searching for literature under an uncommon (nonscientific) name. The scientific classification of animals (taxonomy: genus species) is an important tool that can be used to determine the needs of a particular animal because it provides a "real identity" to the animal. Of course, with over 6,800 different species of reptiles and 4,500 species of amphibians, the task of learning all of these scientific names would be impossible. There are approximately 100 different species that are routinely offered for sale in the pet trade, and individuals working with these animals should develop a resource library to become familiar with both their scientific and common names. The scientific classification of animals is dynamic and may change, so keeping up with new and updated literature is recommended. A list of common scientific and common names can be found in Table 2-1.

HUSBANDRY

ENVIRONMENTAL CONCERNS

Pet reptiles require more attention regarding their husbandry and management than other pets, such as birds, dogs, and cats. Many of the successes and failures experienced by your clients are directly related to their ability to accommodate their pet reptile's nutritional, psychological, and environmental requirements.

The single most important factor to maintaining a healthy reptile in captivity is providing an appropriate environmental temperature range (ETR). Reptiles are ectotherms and depend on their environmental temperature to regulate their core body temperature. Establishing an appropriate ETR for a reptile requires knowledge of the animal's native environment and living habits.

Reptile species are found throughout much of the world's temperate and tropical climates. To survive within these climates, reptiles have adapted to specific niches. An arboreal lizard (such as a green iguana) and a burrowing lizard (such as a skink) from Central America may be found in the same geographic location, but they are exposed to different ETRs because of their different behavioral patterns. A green iguana may experience temperatures greater than 100°F in the trees and 85–90°F in the shade, whereas a subterranean animal may experience temperatures less than 85°F in its burrow. Researching the origin and specific needs of a reptile will improve our ability to care for these animals in captivity.

Table 2-1
Reptile and Amphibian Taxonomy

Class Reptilia
Order Crocodylia   (Alligators, Caimans, Crocodilians, Gharials)
    American alligator   *Alligator mississipiensis*
    American crocodile   *Crocodylus acutus*
    Speckled caiman   *Caiman crocodilus*
Order Chelonia   (Turtles, Tortoises and Terrapins)
    Box turtle   *Terrapene carolina*
    Red-ear slider   *Trachemmys scripta elegans*
    Gopher tortoise   *Gopherus polyphemus*
    Desert tortoise   *Gopherus agassizii*
    Leopard tortoise   *Geochelone pardalis*
    Mata-mata   *Chelus fimbriatus*
    Red-footed tortoise   *Geochelone carbonaria*
    Snapping turtle   *Chelydra serpentina*
    Sulcatta tortoise   *Geochelone sulcatta*
Order Squamata   (Lizards and Snakes)
  Lizards
    Bearded dragon   *Pogonia vitticeps*
    Bosc's (Savannah) monitor   *Varanus exanthematicus*
    Chinese water dragon   *Physignathus lesueri*
    Green anole   *Anolis carolinensis*
    Green plumed basilisk   *Basiliscus plumifrons*
    Green iguana   *Iguana iguana*
    Jackson's chameleon   *Chamaeleo jacksonii*
    Leopard gecko   *Eublepharis macularius*
    Panther chameleon   *Furcifer pardalis*
    Prehensile-tailed skink   *Corucia zebrata*
    Veiled chameleon   *Chamaeleo calyptratus*
  Snakes
    Ball python   *Python regius*
    Boa constrictor   *Boa constrictor constrictor*
    Burmese python   *Python molurus bivittatus*
    Corn snake   *Elaphe guttata guttata*
    Garter snake   *Thamnophis* spp.
    King snake   *Lampropeltis getulus*
    Reticulated python   *Python reticulatus*

Table continued on next page

Table 2-1, cont.
Reptile and Amphibian Taxonomy

Class Amphibia	
Order Anura (Frogs and Toads)	
American bullfrog	*Rana catesbeiana*
African clawed frog	*Xenopus laevis*
Argentine horned frog	*Ceratophrys ornata*
Cane toad	*Bufo marinus*
Leopard frog	*Rana pipiens*
Poison-arrow frog	*Phyllobates* spp., *Dendrobates* spp.
Order Urodela (Salamanders and Newts)	
Axolotl	*Ambystoma mexicanum*
Hellbender	*Cryptobranchus* spp.
Mudpuppy	*Necturus maculatus*
Tiger salamander	*Ambystoma tigrinum*
Order Gymnophiona (Caecilians)	
Aquatic caecilian	*Typhlonectes natans*
Indonesian caecilian	*Ichthyophis kohtaoensis*

Providing an appropriate ETR for a reptile can be accomplished using a number of commercially available products. Recommendations for heating products should be based on the anatomy and natural behaviors of the reptile. For example, the large surface area of the turtle's carapace serves as a heat collection device when the animal basks under radiant light. Therefore, the use of substrate heat sources (e.g., hot rocks, and undertank heating pads) will be of limited value.

The preferred method of providing heat for reptiles is radiant light. Reptiles naturally bask under the radiant light of the sun to store heat, which serves to maintain their core body temperature. Variable wattage incandescent bulbs can be used to provide an appropriate ETR. Always provide a barrier between the light source and the animal to prevent contact with the heat source. Thermometers should be used to measure the temperature and ensure that the ETR is appropriate for that particular species.

Historically, "hot rocks" have been recommended for reptiles, but have been associated with thermal burns. In many cases, the hot rock was the only source of heat for the reptile in its enclosure. Reptiles will gravitate to environmental heat to regulate their core temperature. Many hot rocks can generate excessively high temperatures (>110°F) or "hot spots" that can severely burn an animal. Large reptiles that can actually cover a hot rock can trap the heat and develop a significant burn. This problem is not exclusive to hot rocks. Snakes provided direct contact to an incandescent bulb (e.g., radiant heat) in an environment where the temperature is not regulated have been known to wrap themselves around the bulb and severely burn themselves. The certified veterinary technician should be able to make recommendations for clients that would prevent these disasters from occurring. Newer generation hot rocks are offered for sale and claim not to generate the excessive temperatures observed in the past. Another disadvantage of the hot rock is that it provides only a single point source of heat. Hot rocks have been used successfully with other heat sources (e.g., radiant light) to provide a basking area for "sun-loving" species. Hot rocks should only be used for basking lizards that do not "cover-up" the hot rock. The surface temperature of the hot rock should be monitored closely.

Undertank heating pads are commonly used for snakes and lizards. Undertank heating sources can be placed on one side of an animal's enclosure, leaving the other area unheated. This will effectively provide the animal with an appropriate ETR. When these devices are placed under a glass enclosure, the heat generated can be much higher than on the pad's surface, leading to burns. The temperatures generated by these heating devices should be monitored closely.

The reptile's metabolism, immune system, and behavior are directly related to its ability to maintain its core body temperature. A reptile maintained at an inappropriate ETR will become hypothermic and have a decreased metabolism, resulting in inactivity and limited growth. A reptile with decreased immune function will be unable to mount an effective immune response against bacterial, viral, and fungal pathogens. Many of these animals are classified as "poor-doers." Successful treatment (e.g., antibiotics) of infectious diseases in reptiles requires that the animal be maintained at an appropriate ETR for their metabolism to effectively distribute the medication to the target tissues.

Recommendations for providing a reptile with an appropriate ETR will depend on the species. Radiant light (e.g., incandescent lamps or ceramic heat emitters) most closely resembles the radiant heat generated by the sun that reptiles encounter in the wild.

Full-spectrum lighting has received a great deal of attention in reptile literature because of its role as an "artificial sun" in the management of captive reptiles. The sun naturally produces three types of radiation: ultraviolet (290-400nm), visible (400-700nm), and infrared (>700nm). Ultraviolet radiation can be further divided into ultraviolet A (320-400nm), ultraviolet B (290-320nm), and ultraviolet C (<290nm) wavelengths. Ultraviolet A has been associated with reproductive behaviors in some lizard species. Ultraviolet B plays a role in the endogenous synthesis of vitamin D. An animal that derives its vitamin D_3 from photochemical synthesis, rather than dietary intake, will require regular exposure to ultraviolet B radiation to ensure that it will synthesize adequate levels of vitamin D. Vitamin D serves several functions in the body, including the absorption of calcium at the level of the intestine. There has been limited research to assess the role of ultraviolet B (UVB) in the endogenous synthesis of vitamin D in reptiles, and much of what we know is anecdotal. To ensure that a captive reptile or amphibian is provided the maximal UVB radiation, the bulb should be positioned within 18 inches of the animal and not directed through glass. Glass refracts short-wavelength light, effectively inhibiting UVB radiation penetration. Reptiles should be provided a 12-hour light, 12-hour darkness cycle under normal conditions; however, individuals interested in breeding these animals should establish photoperiods that mimic natural seasonal cycles. Full-spectrum light bulbs should be replaced every 12 months because they lose their effectiveness over time.

Environmental humidity is often overlooked by most pet reptile owners. Most recommendations for relative humidity in captive settings are based on the climate that an animal originates from: tropical 80–95%, temperate 60–70%, and desert 40–50%.[1] Many reptiles are dependent on environmental moisture to aid with shedding and to maintain hydration. When animals are predisposed to low relative humidity, they are prone to dysecdysis (difficulty shedding), dehydration, respiratory infections, and behavioral anomalies. Humidity can be maintained or increased in an enclosure by utilizing large surface area water bowls, bubbling or heating water in a mason jar, covering the enclosure lid with a plastic sheet, and routine misting. A hygrometer should be placed into the cage to closely monitor the relative humidity.

Reptiles have developed various behaviors that enable them to fill a certain niche in their environment. Attempts should be made to provide the animal with "cage furniture" that encourages these behaviors. For example, the green iguana is arboreal (a tree-climber). These animals naturally climb into tree branches to bask under radiant sunlight. When these animals are placed in an enclosure that does not contain branches, they are more likely to be stressed. Stress can initiate a cascade of physiologic changes in the body that can affect the metabolism and immune function. Pet owners should be made aware of the importance of fully researching the specific needs of their new pet and providing them a suitable captive environment. Cage furniture should be safe, non-ingestible, and easy to clean (Figure 2-1).

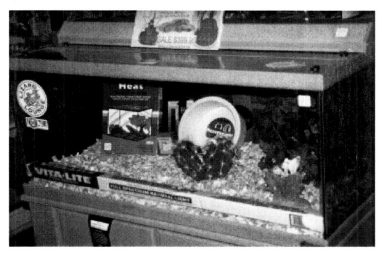

Figure 2-1 Reptile cage and accessories. Providing an appropriate environment is necessary for maintaining a healthy reptile.

There are a number of different substrates available in the pet retail market. Every substrate has potential advantages and disadvantages related to its use (Table 2-2). Recommendations to the owner should always include providing the pet with a substrate that is safe, easy to clean, and aesthetic (Figure 2-2). Substrates should be cleaned regularly; all fecal material and urates should be removed daily to prevent possible contact dermatitis.

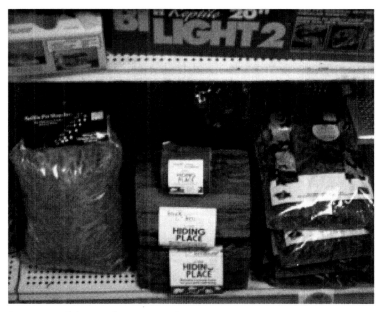

Figure 2-2 Substrates. There are a number of various substrates available to pet owners.

Table 2-2
Substrates Commonly Recommended for Reptiles and Amphibians

Substrate	Advantages	Disadvantages
Newspaper	Inexpensive Easy to clean Easy to monitor feces, urine	Aesthetically unpleasing Affords no cover to reptile
Orchid bark	Aesthetically pleasing Natural	Predisposes to foreign body Reduces relative humidity Dusty (respiratory signs)
Calcium carbonate sand	Aesthetically pleasing Easy to clean	Costly Foreign bodies in eye, mouth
Aspen wood shavings	Aesthetically pleasing Easy to clean	Reduces relative humidity Splinters/foreign bodies

NUTRITION

In the wild, reptiles have the opportunity to select from a diverse array of food items in their environment to meet their daily needs, but with over 11,000 species of reptiles

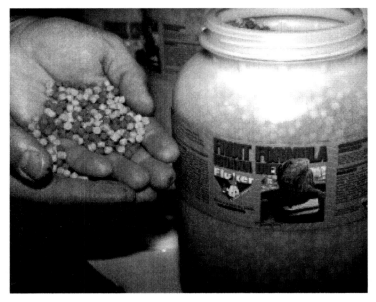

and amphibians in the world it can be difficult to re-create these diets in captivity. By researching the specific dietary requirements of reptiles and amphibians and having an understanding of the nutritional value of commercially available foods, you can educate your clients and ensure their success with managing their pet reptile or amphibian (Figure 2-3).

Figure 2-3 Reptile food. Commercially prepared diets are helpful in meeting the complex nutritional requirements of pets.

Reptile feeding habits can be classified into one of three categories: carnivores, omnivores, and herbivores. Adult amphibians are all carnivorous, while larval forms may be carnivorous (e.g., salamanders) or herbivorous (e.g., tadpoles). Carnivores are the easiest animals to accommodate because they will accept mammals, such as rats and mice, which are a nutritionally balanced food resource. A common mistake that pet owners make when feeding carnivores is to offer live prey. When a reptile is not hungry, it will rarely kill the prey item. If left unattended, the prey will become hungry and feed on the reptile. These attacks can prove fatal. To prevent this from occurring, recommend to your clients that they pre-kill the prey items. Reptiles utilize olfaction to detect their prey items and can easily be trained to eat pre-killed prey.

Another common group of carnivores—the insectivores—feed exclusively on invertebrates. There are six commercially available invertebrates offered for sale, including the domestic cricket (*Acheta domestica*), mealworm (*Tenebrio molitor*), superworm (*Zoophobias morio*), earthworms (*Lumbricus terrestris*), and greater wax moth larva (*Galleria mellonella*) (Figure 2-4). These commercial invertebrates are often offered for sale and are not nutritionally prepared. All living creatures require energy, and if feeder invertebrates are not offered food, they will provide little nutritional value to the reptile. Commercially available invertebrates are adequate in protein and fat, but are deficient in specific amino acids, vitamins, and minerals. The most common nutritional disorder

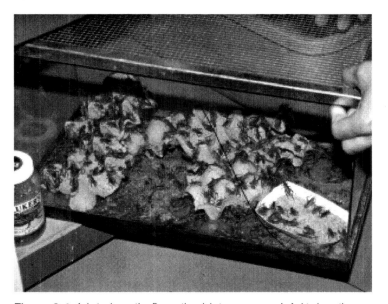

observed in insectivores is secondary nutritional hyperparathyroidism. A rapidly growing insectivore, such as a leopard gecko, will develop muscle tremors, seizures, and possible death when offered a calcium-deficient diet. This problem can be prevented by properly preparing the feeder invertebrate. Many pet retailers offer invertebrates an apple or potato,

Figure 2-4 *Acheta domestica.* Domestic crickets are commonly fed to insectivores.

believing that they are offering the prey items a balanced diet. These food items provide little more than carbohydrates and moisture and do not solve the mineral deficiency of the feeder invertebrate. A solution to this problem is to offer a balanced commercial invertebrate diet. Research evaluating these diets has proven that they can significantly improve the nutritional value of the prey item.[2] Recommend that your clients offer the commercial diet for a minimum of 24 hours prior to offering the prey items to the reptile. This should ensure that the invertebrate will be "gut-loaded." There are also mineral supplements that can be used to "dust" the prey items and increase their nutritional value. These mineral supplements should be used according to label recommendations.

Herbivores are the hardest group of reptiles to accommodate in captivity because of the limited commercial availability of quality commercial vegetables and fruits. In the wild, herbivorous reptiles select their diet from a variety of available resources, whereas in captivity we are limited to what is available.

The greens most frequently recommended as the base diet for captive herbivores are romaine lettuce and mustard and collard greens. Other plant products such as spinach, broccoli, green beans, kale, squash, dandelion leaves, and other dark leafy vegetables can be used to further diversify the diet. Certain plant products, such as kale and spinach, should be limited in the diet because they contain oxalates and can bind valuable dietary calcium in the digestive tract and increase the likelihood of a mineral deficiency.[3] Other plant products, such as broccoli, contain goitrogens which can alter thyroid metabolism and should likewise be limited. The key to success with herbivore diets is to provide a diverse selection of food products to increase the nutritional value offered to the animal. Fruits should not constitute more than 10–15% of the animals diet because they are devoid of protein and essential minerals.

In recent years, commercial herbivore diets have been manufactured that improve our ability to provide a more balanced diet. Many of these diets are marketed as complete and recommended as a sole source of nutrition; however, little is known about reptile nutrition and a more diverse diet should be recommended. A diet that combines a commercial product (25–40%) mixed with high quality plant sources, such as romaine lettuce, mustard and collard greens, may be used.

There are a number of commercially available nutritional supplements for reptiles and amphibians. The available supplements may contain calcium, calcium and phosphorus, vitamins, amino acids, and a combination of these nutrients. Little is known regarding the specific dietary requirements of reptiles and amphibians. In the past, many of the nutritional problems diagnosed in reptiles and amphibians were associated with vitamin and mineral deficiencies and the need for supplements was apparent. More recently, diseases associated with excessive vitamin and mineral supplements have been reported and a concern has arisen regarding how much to provide these animals.[4] Clients should be made aware of the risks of vitamin and mineral over-supplementation. A veterinarian should make specific dietary recommendations based upon the reptile's or amphibian's age and physiologic status (e.g., gravid).

TRANSPORT

Reptiles can elicit quite an array of emotions in people. Clients with dogs or cats may not appreciate sharing a waiting room with a large reptile. To prevent potential disaster in your veterinary hospital, recommend that reptile and amphibian owners transport their pets in a closed, secured enclosure. Snakes and lizards travel well in ventilated burlap or cotton bags. Larger snakes, lizards, and tortoises may be transported in large plastic boxes or garbage cans with air holes. Semi-aquatic reptiles (e.g., red-ear slider turtles) and amphibians (e.g., bullfrog) should be transported in a plastic box (with air holes) with a water level that covers the animal's feet. Semi-aquatic animals maintained in deep water for transport are prone to drowning. Totally aquatic amphibians (e.g., Surinam frog) should be transported in a plastic enclosure with sufficient dechlorinated water to cover the animal. Recommend to your clients that they not change the bedding of the enclosure so that the fecal and urine material can be examined.

HISTORY

A thorough history is essential to making an appropriate diagnosis for any exotic animal case because many of the problems identified in exotic animals are directly related to inappropriate husbandry. A veterinary technician should first collect the signalment, including age, breed, and gender if it is known. Knowledge of the animal's age and gender can be useful when developing a differential diagnosis list. For example, an adult intact female green iguana with a history of weakness and lethargy during the months of December through March may be suffering from a reproductive problem (e.g., follicular stasis or dystocia), whereas an adult male would not.

After collecting the signalment, the history should focus on background information, including where the animal was acquired, length of time owned, if the client has other pets or reptiles, if he recently acquired another animal, and the interaction between the owner and his pet (e.g., frequency of handling, if any). This information should provide the technician with an initial understanding of the client's knowledge of his pet reptile.

The next set of questions should focus on how the animal is managed at home (husbandry), including: whether the animal is housed indoors or outdoors; if it has supervised or unsupervised run in the house; the cage size and material; the cage location in the house; temperature, humidity, lighting, light cycle, and substrate used in the cage; types of cage furniture; if the reptile is housed with another animal; and how often the cage is cleaned and the type of disinfectant. Questions about the animal's nutrition are also important and should include type of food (natural or commercial), amount offered daily, frequency, supplements, water source, and how often the food and water are changed.

Finally, the questions should focus on the animal's current health status and questions should include past medical history, current presenting problem, and the duration of the complaint. Although it is natural to want to focus on the problem at hand first, a great deal of information may be lost if the history is not collected in a thorough and systematic approach.

RESTRAINT

Handling an animal for an examination using appropriate techniques is essential to protect yourself, the veterinarian, the client, and the patient. A working knowledge of the animal's anatomy and physiology are important considerations. First, determine what weapons the animal may use to defend itself. For example, a green iguana may use its tail to "whip" you, its teeth to bite, and its claws to climb away or on you. Identifying these weapons prior to grasping and "man-handling" the animal will result in a reduced likelihood of injury for you and your patient. Reptiles and amphibians lack a diaphragm. If these animals are grasped tightly around the rib cage, you can literally suffocate them. Chelonians should never be held upside down for extended periods because the viscera can place extra pressure on the lungs, again leading to difficulty breathing. Appropriate training and practice will enable you to safely manage a wide range of nonvenomous reptiles.

LIZARDS

For small specimens, place your thumb and index finger on each side of the ramus (mandible) and allow the animal's body to rest in the palm of your hand (Figure 2-5). Never constrict the animal's body when you are restraining it because reptiles, except crocodilians, lack a diaphragm and you can suffocate them. For larger specimens, again place your index finger and thumb on the corners of the mandible and use your second hand to hold the rear legs against the tail. Never grab a lizard by the tail. Some species (e.g., green iguana) have the ability to "drop" their tail. This is a defense mechanism which allows an animal to avoid capture by a predator. Clients are not impressed when their pet lizard's tail is broken because of poor restraint technique.

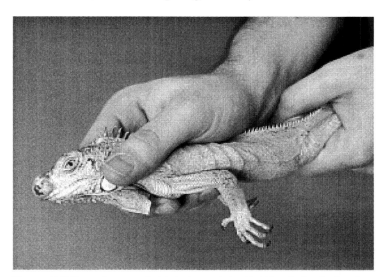

Figure 2-5 Proper iguana restraint. An iguana is best held by placing the thumb and forefinger of one hand around the mandible, while using the other hand to secure the legs to the tail.

SNAKES

Place your index finger and thumb under the mandible and use your additional hand to support the body (Figure 2-6). One person is required for every 2–3 feet of snake. Large constrictor species should never be handled without assistance. Although rare, these large, powerful snakes are capable of seriously injuring an individual who is careless. Only trained professionals should ever handle venomous snakes, and access to anti-venom should be arranged at a local hospital.

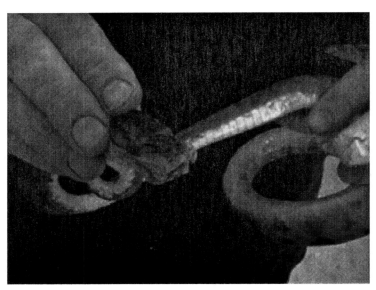

Figure 2-6 Proper snake restraint. A snake can be held by securing the head with one hand and using the other hand to support the body.

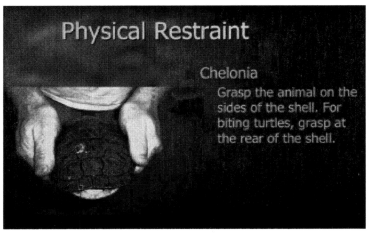

Physical Restraint

Chelonia

Grasp the animal on the sides of the shell. For biting turtles, grasp at the rear of the shell.

Figure 2-7A Proper turtle restraint grasping the sides of the shell.

CHELONIANS

Most chelonians can be handled by grasping the middle of the shell (Figure 2-7A). Many of the biting turtles (e.g., snapping turtles) should be grasped at the rear of the shell. For a physical examination, the head and neck can be gently withdrawn from the shell (Figure 2-7B). Do not exert excessive force when restraining them because you could easily damage their cervical spine. In those cases where the animal cannot be physically managed, an appropriate sedative or anesthetic can be provided by the veterinarian.

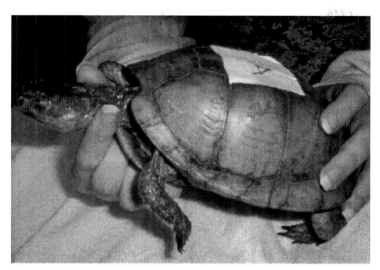

Figure 2-7B Proper turtle restraint (holding the head of the turtle and rear of the shell) to facilitate the examination of the head.

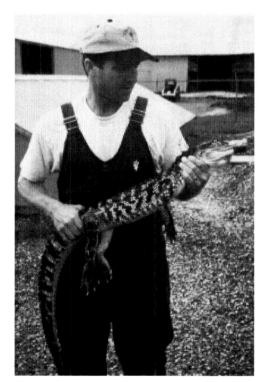

Figure 2-8 Proper alligator restraint. An alligator can be held in the same fashion as smaller specimens, but duct tape may be used to close the mouth.

CROCODILIANS

Crocodilians are lightning fast and can inflict a nasty bite. They should be restrained only by experienced professionals. Crocodilians have very powerful muscles to close their jaws, but the muscles to open the jaws are not as powerful. A crocodilian should be grasped around the neck, the mouth pushed closed and taped with "duct tape." Once the mouth is appropriately restricted, a crocodilian can be restrained in a manner similar to that described for large lizard specimens (Figure 2-8).

AMPHIBIANS

Amphibians have a very delicate and sensitive epidermis. The epidermis is covered by a protective mucous barrier, similar to that of fish, which defends these animals against pathogens. There are also amphibians, such as poison-dart frogs, that produce toxins in these mucous secretions. To prevent danger to yourself and the animal, wear a pair of latex examination gloves that have been moistened with dechlorinated water or distilled water to prevent damage to the animal's protective mucous barrier and toxic exposure to the handler. Large amphibians (e.g., Argentine horned frogs, and hellbenders) can inflict a nasty bite and precautions should be taken when managing these large specimens. Most amphibians can be grasped in the palm of the hand and examined. Some salamanders can detach their tail, as described with lizards, and should never be grasped by the tail.

PHYSICAL EXAMINATION

The physical examination of a reptile or amphibian will relay a great deal of information to the veterinarian and guide in diagnosis. Reptiles and amphibians have evolved to mask their illnesses to prevent predation. Therefore, a "hands-off" examination of the animal in its enclosure should be performed before a routine "hands-on" examination. Closely observe the animal's general disposition, respiratory rate, and locomotion. Record your findings and proceed to a "hands-on" examination.

Always perform a "hands-on" physical examination in a thorough and consistent manner. There are some individuals who prefer to start at the head and work their way back, while others start from the tail and work to the head. A basic understanding of what is normal for that animal is also an important prerequisite. For example, chameleons typically have bright yellow mucous membranes. If you did not realize this, you might misclassify this animal as being icteric. Maintain a resource library that will allow you to identify particular differences between species.

The eyes should be clear and free of discharge. The nares and external ears (tympanum in chelonians and amphibians, absent in snakes) should be free of discharge and ectoparasites (e.g., ticks and mites). Some reptiles possess salt glands in the nares that may produce a clear, crystalline secretion.

The oral cavity should be opened with care because aggressive manipulation can lead to broken teeth, beak (chelonians), or damage to the mucous membranes. A rubber spatula or folded piece of radiographic film may be gently inserted into the mouth of a lizard or snake to visualize the oral cavity. A paperclip may be used to gently pry open the jaws of a chelonian. Aggressive reptiles may gape as a defensive or offensive measure, which will facilitate an examination of the oral cavity. The oral cavity should be clear and free of discharge, parasites, and abscesses. The mucous membranes should be moist and pale-pink in color. The glottis (airway) should be examined for discharge and parasites.

The skin should be clean and free of defects. Imported animals are often covered with ectoparasites and should be examined closely, especially in the gular fold (under the chin), mouth, and around the eyes. The limbs should be checked for range of motion and palpated for any skeletal deformities. The coelomic cavity should be palpated and assessed for pain and abnormal masses. The internal organs of reptiles and amphibians are consistent across species; therefore, a basic understanding of reptilian and amphibian anatomy will be necessary to interpret abnormal findings. In some amphibians, such as frogs, a penlight can be held up to the animal's skin on the lateral body wall to view the internal organs.

A physical examination should include auscultation of the animal's heart and lungs. Auscultation in reptiles is especially difficult because the scales can inhibit your ability to fully assess the heart and lung fields. A thin, damp paper towel can be placed on the skin of the animal to reduce the friction caused between the bell of the stethoscope and the scales. Even when this technique is used the heart and lungs may not be heard. Although reptiles are difficult to auscult, we highly recommend being thorough and consistent with every patient. An ultrasonic doppler may also be used to monitor the heart rate of a reptile or amphibian.

DIAGNOSTIC SAMPLING

Veterinarians use the information gathered from a detailed history and thorough physical examination to develop a list of differential diagnoses. The veterinarian will then use available diagnostic tests—such as hematology, plasma chemistry analysis, radiographs, microbiological isolation, cytologic examination, and parasitologic examination—to determine the cause of the animal's illness.

BLOOD WORK

Reptiles and amphibians mask their illness, making diagnosis difficult. Hematologic sampling provides a veterinarian with insight into possible physiologic changes and the disease status of an animal. Samples are routinely collected and submitted to evaluate the red and white blood cells (complete blood count), plasma enzymes, and electrolytes. The volume of blood that can be safely collected from a reptile is 0.5–0.8% of its body weight or 0.5–0.8-ml/100g body weight.[5] It is important to consider the animal's history and physical examination when determining the volume of blood that can be collected. An animal that has experienced an acute blood loss (e.g., trauma) cannot afford to have large volumes of blood collected. Fortunately, most laboratories can perform a CBC and a plasma chemistry analysis on approximately 1-ml of blood.

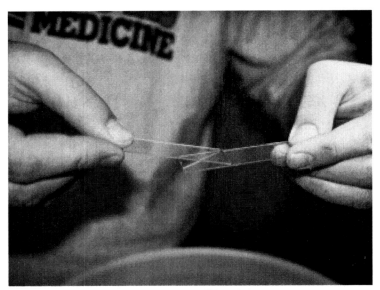

Figure 2-9A Blood smear using the glass slide technique.

Blood samples should be collected using heparinized needles and placed into appropriate collection tubes immediately after sample collection. Laboratories may vary in their preference for collection tubes, so it is recommended to contact them prior to sample submission. Lizard and snake blood samples submitted for hematologic examination may be placed into a vial with EDTA (ethylenediaminetetracetic acid: purple-top) or lithium heparin (green top). Chelonian blood samples should always be placed into a vial with lithium heparin, rather than EDTA, to prevent blood cell anomalies. Blood samples collected for plasma chemistry analysis should be placed into a vial with lithium heparin.

When reptile and amphibian blood smears are prepared using mammalian techniques (e.g., slide smear), the cells may be damaged or distorted, making interpretation difficult. The addition of 1 drop of 22 % bovine albumin (Gamma Biologicals, Inc, Houston, TX, 77092) to 5 drops of blood appears to stabilize the cell membranes and improve cell visualization. The slide smear technique is similar to that described for mammals. A drop of blood is placed on the end of a clean, dust-free slide. The end of a second slide is placed in front of the blood droplet on a 45° angle and drawn back until the blood spreads across the surface of the end of the slide (Figure 2-9A). A smooth, rapid "push" forward will spread the blood across the slide. The blood smear should have a

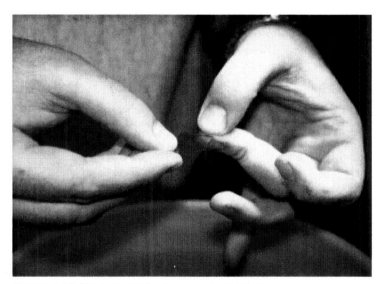

Figure 2-9B Blood smear using the cover slip technique.

feathered edge. Another technique, the cover-slip technique, can be performed by placing a drop of blood on to a clean, dust-free cover slip. A second cover slip is rotated at a 90° angle and placed on top of the first cover slip (Figure 2-9B). As the blood spreads between the two cover slips, the top piece is pulled away and there should be a well-defined feathered edge. The cover slip is fragile and precautions should be taken to prevent breakage during the staining process. The cover slip must be placed on to a slide to facilitate interpreting the sample on a microscope and should be secured using glue to prevent loss of the cover slip.

In many hospitals, a licensed veterinary technician may be asked to perform white blood cell counts. There are several different techniques that can be used to perform a white blood cell count, including the Unopette #5877 system (Becton-Dickinson) and a white blood cell estimate. The commercial system should be performed following the manufacturer's instructions. A white blood cell estimate can be performed at any veterinary hospital with a microscope, slides, and stains. White blood cell estimates are not as exact as the Unopette system, but provide the veterinarian with insight into the animal's condition. A white blood cell smear can be stained using a Diff-Quick (American Scientific Products, McGraw Park, IL), Giemsa or Wright's stain. The slide should be evaluated on low power (4–10x) to ascertain the quality of the slide preparation. The estimate should be performed on high dry power (45x). The estimate is performed by reviewing 10 different fields of evenly distributed cells. The total number of cells identified from the 10 fields should be divided by 10 to get an average. The average number can then be multiplied by 2,000 to determine the white blood cell estimate. After the white blood cell estimate is completed, a differential to determine the representative white blood cells should be performed. The primary white blood cell types in reptiles include the heterophil, lymphocyte, monocyte, eosinophil, azurophil, and basophil. With the exception of the heterophil, the white blood cells are similar in appearance and function to mammalian white blood cells. The heterophil is considered analogous to the mammalian neutrophil; however, its appearance and function are slightly different. The reptilian and amphibian heterophil possesses a round to oval nucleus and red-orange rod-shaped granules. The heterophil will often be misinterpreted as an eosinophil by a beginner.

BLOOD COLLECTION

Lizards

Blood samples are routinely collected from the ventral coccygeal vein or ventral abdominal vein in lizards. The ventral tail vein is located on the ventral midline of the tail. The blood sample should be collected from within the proximal 1/4 of the tail. When a sample from an adult male animal is required, one should avoid the hemipenes by collecting the sample distal to the hemipenal bulges. Clean the venipuncture site with an appropriate disinfectant to remove any excess organic debris. A 22–25-gauge needle fastened to a 3-ml syringe should be used to collect the sample. For large animals, a longer needle (1.5–2") may be required to collect the sample. The needle should be inserted perpendicular to the skin and inserted to the point of the caudal vertebrae (Figure 2-10A). Gently apply negative pressure as the needle-syringe is withdrawn off of the caudal vertebrae. In some cases, the venipuncturist must "walk the bone" to identify the blood vessel. Always be conscientious of your patient when collecting a sample and be as "quick and kind" as possible. Some lizard species have tail autonomy as a defense mechanism against predators and will drop their tail if handled inappropriately.

The ventral abdominal vein is located on the ventral midline within the body cavity. This site is routinely used, but the tail is the preferred site. (However, there have been a few reported instances of individuals lacerating the ventral abdominal vein, only to have the animal die later from bleeding out.) The site should be aseptically prepared. Again, a 22–25-gauge needle fastened to a 3-ml syringe should be used. The bevel of the needle should face up and the needle inserted at an approximately 15–30° angle, practically parallel to the body wall (Figure 2-10B). Negative pressure should be applied once the needle is inserted. Do not "fish around" performing this technique; being overly aggressive can lead to visceral damage. The toenail has also been recommended, in some books, as a site of blood collection in lizards; however, the blood collected from these sites is often diluted with lymph and is of little value.

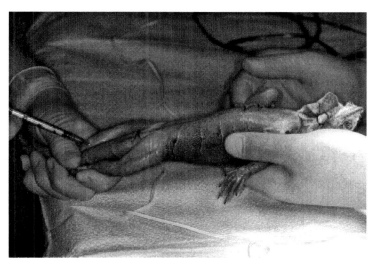

Figure 2-10A Lizard venipuncture. Blood collection via the ventral tail vein.

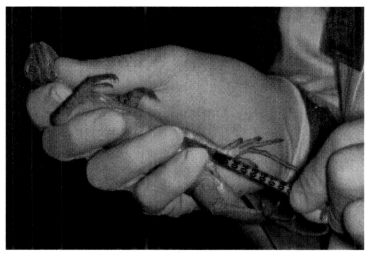

Figure 2-10B Blood collection via the ventral abdominal vein in a lizard.

Chelonians

Blood samples are routinely collected from the jugular vein, dorsal coccygeal sinus, or brachial vein. Blood collection in chelonians may require sedation if the animal does not tolerate restraint of its head or limbs. Placing excess strain on the neck or limbs during restraint can lead to broken cervical vertebrae or limbs. A 22–25-gauge needle fastened to a 3-ml syringe can be used to collect blood samples at any of the prescribed sites. The venipuncture sites should be aseptically prepared to remove any excess organic debris. The right jugular vein is generally more prominent than the left and is located on the lateral aspect of the neck, approximately at the level of the tympanum (ear). An assistant should gently retract the head to facilitate exposure. An index finger should be placed on the neck to assist with jugular vein visualization. In some cases, the jugular vein cannot be visualized and a "blind-stick" is attempted (Figure 2-11A).

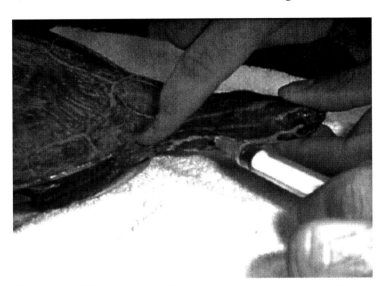

Figure 2-11A Turtle venipuncture. The jugular vein is being used for the collection of blood.

The brachial vein is located on the posterior aspect of the elbow. This venipuncture site has been used with great success with tortoises and can be performed without sedation. An assistant should withdraw the leg and place one or more fingers proximal to the elbow to facilitate exposure. The needle should be inserted perpendicular to the posterior aspect of the elbow and negative pressure applied immediately after penetrating the skin (Figure 2-11B). This venipuncture site is often a "blind-stick." One drawback of this site is that the brachial vein is closely associated with lymph and a diluted or "mixed" sample is collected that cannot be used for hematologic evaluation. A diluted or mixed sample will looked "watered-down" or thin.

The dorsal coccygeal sinus is located on the dorsal midline of the tail. The tail should be extended and a 25-gauge needle inserted on the dorsal midline in a cranial direction (Figure 2-11C). Again, this site is closely associated with lymph and a mixed sample may be collected.

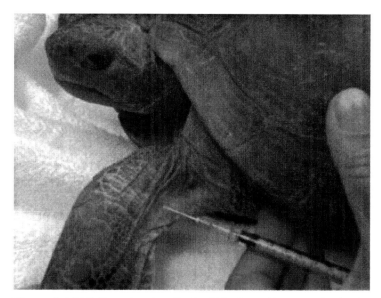

Figure 2-11B Turtle venipuncture. The brachial vein provides a route for blood collection in the turtle.

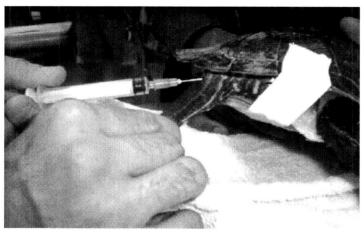

Figure 2-11C Turtle venipuncture. The dorsal coccygeal sinus can also be employed in blood collection.

Snakes

Blood samples are routinely collected from the heart, ventral coccygeal vein, and palatine veins. Cardiocentesis is the preferred method and provides large volumes of blood if necessary. The heart is located approximately 1/3 to 1/4 the distance from the head. This procedure is routinely performed on snakes over 200 grams without sedation. It is essential that there is enough assistance to restrain the snake during the procedure to prevent injury to itself and the handlers. The animal should be positioned on its dorsum and the heart localized by visual inspection or palpation. Snakes are quite capable of moving their heart cranially or caudally, so it is important to "immobilize" it by inserting an index finger cranial to the heart and the thumb caudal to the heart. A 22–25-gauge needle of variable length, based on snake size, should be inserted under the scale at

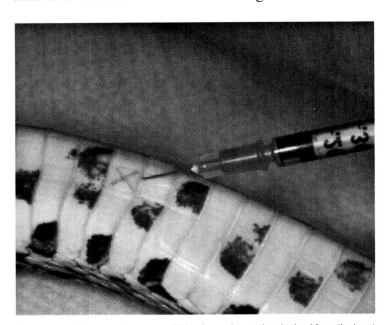

Figure 2-12 Snake venipuncture. A blood sample may be obtained from the heart of a snake.

the most distal point of the beating heart (ventricle) (Figure 2-12). Apply negative pressure once the needle is inserted. The blood will literally be pumped into the syringe with each heartbeat.

The ventral coccygeal vein is located on the ventral midline of the tail. Collection of blood from this site is usually possible only in larger snakes. The snake's body should be supported by a set of hands per 3–4 feet of body length. The tail should be grasped by the individual collecting the sample. The sample should be collected in the proximal 1/3 of the tail. Care should be taken not to damage the hemipenes of a male by staying on the midline. A 22–25-gauge needle should be inserted at a 45° angle under a ventral scale and advanced to the caudal vertebrae. Negative pressure should be applied and the needle retracted until blood is visualized in the hub of the needle.

The palatine vessels are located on the dorsal palate inside of the mouth. Intravenous catheters can be placed in these vessels in larger nonvenomous snakes. The oral cavity should be opened using an appropriate speculum. The palatine vessels are located between the palatine and maxillary teeth. A 25–26-gauge needle should be used for blood collection. The oral cavity is a contaminated environment, so aseptic preparation of the site is difficult. The needle should be inserted into the blood vessel at a 45° angle and negative pressure applied immediately. This location should only be used as a last resort.

Amphibians

Blood samples can be collected in amphibians from the ventral abdominal vein, ventral coccygeal vein, and lingual plexus. Restraining an amphibian for blood collection can be tricky because the animals can be quite slippery. The assistant and individual collecting the samples should wear moistened latex gloves to prevent damaging the animal's skin. A 25–27-gauge needle fastened to a 3-ml syringe should be used for blood collection in amphibians. One should expect increased cellular destruction using the smaller gauge needle. The needle should be heparinized prior to blood collection to prevent clotting.

The ventral abdominal vein is often readily visible in larger amphibians by direct visualization or placing a flashlight near the lateral body wall. Blood collection techniques are similar to that described for lizards.

Blood can be collected from the ventral coccygeal vein in larger salamanders and newts. The approach to this vein is similar to that described in lizards. Some salamanders and newts, like lizards, have tail autonomy and can drop their tail as a natural defense mechanism if handled inappropriately.

The lingual plexus can be used for larger amphibians. The lingual plexus is a complex of blood vessels located under the fleshy tongue. A soft, rubber speculum should be used to gently open the animal's mouth. The skeletons of these animals are fragile in comparison to reptiles and special care should be taken to prevent fractures. Once the mouth is open, a cotton-tip applicator can be used to displace the tongue and facilitate exposure to the venous plexus. A needle (with no syringe attached) can be inserted into the venous plexus and blood can be collected out of the hub of the needle using a microhematocrit tube. Sample contamination from saliva and food material in the oral cavity are likely when using this technique.[6]

MICROBIOLOGY

Bacteria are ubiquitous in the environment. These organisms are commonly differentiated by staining characteristics using a Gram stain (positive or negative) and can be further differentiated based on their biochemical needs: aerobic or anaerobic, lactose fermenting or nonlactose-fermenting, etc. Both Gram-positive and Gram-negative bacteria have been associated with infections in reptiles and amphibians, although opportunistic Gram-negative bacteria are more commonly isolated. Reptiles and amphibians are ectotherms and their core body temperature is regulated based on their environmental temperature and behavioral activities (e.g., basking). Most commercial microbiologic incubators are set at 37°C because they were developed to grow pathogenic bacteria from humans. Because reptile core body temperatures may vary from this standard (37°C), it has been suggested that different temperatures should be used to isolate bacteria from reptiles and amphibians. Unfortunately, establishing an incubator temperature that parallels a reptile's body temperature would be difficult. One possible solution would be to place one sample in a 37°C incubator and another at the animal's body temperature to accommodate organisms that thrive at lower temperature. Regardless of the technique selected, one should always consider a negative culture from a contaminated wound as a possible result of our inability to provide the organism an appropriate temperature.

RADIOLOGY

Radiographs serve as an important diagnostic tool in reptile and amphibian medicine. Radiographs are routinely used to assess a variety of health conditions in these animals, including reproductive (e.g., dystocia), skeletal (e.g., fracture), gastrointestinal (e.g., foreign body), renal (e.g., renomegaly), and respiratory (e.g., pneumonia) problems. Standard safety protocols should be employed when radiographing reptiles and amphibians. The animal may need to be anesthetized for the procedure, although some animals will remain still if placed in a darkened room. A radiographic technique chart should be established based upon a facility's radiographic machine. A high capacity radiographic unit capable of producing 300-milliampere exposures at times of at least 1/60th of a second is recommended. The kVp settings should be adjustable by increments of 2 to provide finite detail. A thorough understanding of reptile and amphibian anatomy is essential to radiographic interpretation.

PARASITOLOGY

Endoparasites

Endoparasites are a common finding in reptiles and amphibians. The same groups of endoparasites commonly identified in domestic species are also routinely identified in reptiles and amphibians, including protozoa, nematodes, trematodes, and cestodes. The majority of reptiles presented to veterinary hospitals are imported and should be considered to have parasites until proven otherwise. Animals and parasites have evolved to "live together," even though the parasite steals nutrition from the host. In captivity, when a reptile or amphibian is exposed to the stress of an inadequate environment and diet, parasites can become more problematic. Parasites will continue to acquire energy from the host, regardless of the host's change in appetite. In these cases, the parasites can become life-threatening. A fecal examination should be performed to identify potential parasites so that an appropriate treatment can be initiated. A fecal saline direct smear and a fecal flotation should be performed on all fecal samples. The direct smear will enable the reviewer to identify bacteria and protozoa, while the fecal float is used to identify larger parasite ova (e.g., roundworms). A fecal examination should always be repeated in 2 weeks, and again in 4 weeks, to determine if the animal is really negative (because shedding can be transient). There are a number of treatment protocols that have been established for treating parasites in reptiles and amphibians (Table 2-3).

Ectoparasites

Imported reptiles routinely have ectoparasites, such as mites, ticks and leeches. These parasites survive by ingesting blood meals from their host. Heavily parasitized juvenile animals can develop a life-threatening anemia. Many of these ectoparasites also serve as vectors for other diseases, including bacterial and possibly viral infections.[7] The diagnosis of an ectoparasite infestation can be made during a thorough physical examination. Leeches are readily identifiable on aquatic reptiles and amphibians. These large ectoparasites should be grasped with forceps and gently separated from the host. The open lesion where the leech was attached should be cleaned and disinfected (e.g., 0.5% chlorhexidine). Ticks are typically not as large as leeches, but are readily identified on external examination. There are three primary life stages of the tick: larva, nymph, and adult. The nymphal and adult stages are differentiated from the larval stages based on the number of appendages (larval: 6, nymphal and adult: 8). The tick burrows its mouthparts into the host to facilitate feeding. Tick removal can be accomplished by grasping the mouthparts where they insert into the host and pulling them out perpendicular to the reptile's skin. Once the parasite is removed it should be properly disposed of. Mites are the smallest of the ectoparasites (1–2mm) and can be easily overlooked. The mite can be found anywhere on the reptile host, although they tend to accumulate around the eyes,

Table 2-3
Antiparasitic Agents used in Reptiles and Amphibians

Drug	Dose	Comments
Fenbendazole	50–100 mg/kg PO Repeat in 7–14 prn	Nematodes[21]
Ivermectin	0.2 mg/kg IM, SC	Nematodes[22] NEVER USE IN CHELONIANS
	5 mg/L water	Topical spray to treat mites[23]
Levamisole	10–20 mg/kg	Nematodes[24]
Metronidazole	40–100 mg/kg PO Repeat 2 weeks	Protozoa[22] Uracoan rattler, milk snakes, tricolor king snakes, and indigo snakes at 40 mg/kg
Praziquantel	5–8 mg/kg IM, SC	Cestodes and trematodes[25]

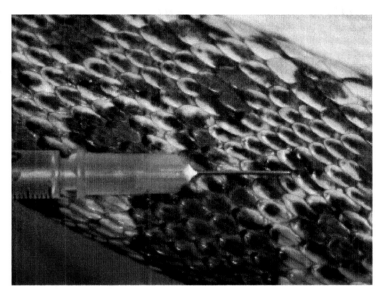

Figure 2-13A Therapeutics. An intramuscular injection is being administered to a snake.

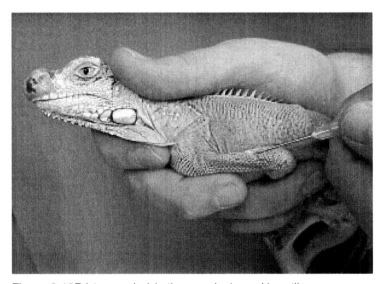

Figure 2-13B Intramuscular injections can also be used in reptiles.

mouth, and gular fold (snakes). A cotton-tip applicator soaked in mineral oil can be used to remove a mite to confirm the diagnosis. The treatment protocols for ectoparasites vary (Table 2-3). Neither ivermectin nor its derivatives should be given to chelonians, as it may be fatal.

THERAPEUTICS

There are no approved therapeutics for reptiles in the United States. Routes of administration for therapeutics and fluids, include per os (PO), subcutaneous (SC), intramuscular (IM), intraosseus (IO), intracoelomic (ICO) and intravenous (IV) (Figures 2-13A and 2-13B). Animals that are in critical condition require routes of administration that provide rapid drug delivery, such as IM, IO or IV, whereas less critical animals may be given therapeutics PO or SC.

Intravenous injections should be administered through an intravenous catheter. The preferred site for intravenous catheterization in chelonians, lizards, and snakes is the jugular vein. The cephalic vein may also be used in lizards.

Intramuscular injections are routinely administered into the epaxial muscles along the spine or in the large muscle groups in the front limbs. Reptiles and amphibians have a renal portal system that may be affected by drug administration in the tail or rear limbs. To avoid these complications, always administer medications in the cranial one-half of the body. The muscle masses of the reptile and amphibian limbs are relatively small in comparison to those of mammals; therefore, injections should be performed sparingly and injection sites (e.g., right leg, left leg) should be alternated.

Reptiles and amphibians are difficult to pill. There are a number of commercial compounding pharmacies that can compound a therapeutic into a liquid and simplify administration.

SURGICAL AND ANESTHETIC ASSISTANCE

Anesthesia and analgesia are relatively new concepts in reptile and amphibian medicine. Only a decade ago, individuals "anesthetized" reptiles by placing them in a refrigerator or freezer to severely restrict their metabolism. This technique should never be used because it does not provide the animal consistent anesthesia or analgesia and can prove fatal. Prior to any anesthetic procedure, the animal should be assessed and determined to be stable. Basic health monitoring should include evaluating the hydration status, heart and respiratory rates, and baseline blood work.

The anesthetics and analgesics used for domestic species (e.g., dogs and cats) are routinely used in reptiles and amphibians, including the dissociatives, propofol, and inhalant anesthetics. The most common dissociatives used in reptile and amphibian anesthesia are ketamine (Ketaset, Fort Dodge Laboratories, Ft. Dodge, IA, USA) and tiletamine plus zolazepam (Telazol, Fort Dodge Laboratories, Ft. Dodge, IA, USA). Ketamine has been used successfully in reptiles and amphibians. Recommended doses vary with reptile and amphibian order, health status, and size of the animal. A dose of 20–40mg/kg ketamine can be given for short painless procedures or as a pre-anesthetic to facilitate intubation. In most species, the animals will be induced within 10–20 minutes. Ketamine provides little to no analgesia, therefore a pre-operative and postoperative analgesic should be considered for painful procedures. A dose of 55–88 mg/kg has been recommended for surgical anesthesia, but ketamine alone should not be considered an adequate surgical anesthetic in these species.[8] There have been a number of side effects reported with ketamine use, including respiratory arrest, bradycardia, and prolonged recovery (1–4 days). Many of these side effects are associated with the administration of high doses (>100 mg/kg), but they can also occur at lower doses. Many anesthetic complications can be prevented by properly evaluating the animal prior to a procedure and monitoring the animal closely during the procedure. Tiletamine is a more potent dissociative agent that is combined with zolazepam to provide muscle relaxation and an anticonvulsant. Tiletamine has been used in snakes and crocodilians with some success, but recoveries are still prolonged. Tiletamine, like ketamine, should not be used for surgical anesthesia in reptiles, but as an induction agent in combination with an inhalant anaesthetic. A dose of 3–5 mg/kg is routinely used with good results.

Propofol has gained in popularity with reptile veterinarians because it provides general anesthesia with a rapid recovery. The primary disadvantage of propofol is that it must be administered intravenously, which can be difficult in smaller specimens. An intravenous butterfly catheter can be used to administer boluses to an animal as the procedure warrants. A dose of 10–14 mg/kg IV in lizards and snakes provides reasonable general anesthesia for 15–30 minutes.[9] A dose of 12–15 mg/kg IV is recommended for chelonians.[9]

Inhalant anesthetics have reduced many of the risks associated with injectable anesthetics. Unlike injectable anesthetics (e.g., ketamine), which cannot be controlled once administered, delivery of an inhalant anesthetic through a precision vaporizer can be controlled based on need. Animals under general inhalant anesthetics should be intubated. Endotracheal tubes ensure that the appropriate anesthetic and oxygen rates are being administered. In the case of an emergency, such as respiratory arrest, valuable time attempting to intubate an animal is not wasted. Endotracheal tube sizes will vary with the order and size of the animals. Chelonians and crocodilians have closed tracheal rings, like birds, and should not have their endotracheal cuff over-inflated. The majority of reptile and amphibian cases presented into private practice are animals under 5 kg and can be maintained using a non-rebreathing system. When a procedure on a larger animal (>5kg) is required, a circle system, similar to that used in dogs, can be used.

The most common inhalants used in veterinary practice are halothane and isoflurane, and both of these anesthetics have been used successfully in reptiles and amphibians. Our knowledge about the metabolism of these gases in reptiles and amphibians is limited and often related to our knowledge in mammals. The elimination of halothane is suspected to occur through liver metabolism and the respiratory system, whereas isoflurane is eliminated exclusively through the respiratory system. Geriatric or compromised cases should be anesthetized using isoflurane because it is unaffected by liver function. There are two trains of thought when anesthetizing an exotic animal:

1. "full-throttle" and

2. incremental anesthesia

The "full-throttle" approach is based on the desire to deliver a high percentage of anesthesia immediately. Many veterinarians will turn the vaporizer directly to 5%. This method is often used to induce fractious animals, because they are anesthetized sooner, and it also delivers high doses to animals that hold their breath. The disadvantage of this technique is that the animal can become deeply anesthetized and, if not monitored closely, they can become apneic and die. The recommended approach is to deliver an inhalant anesthetic in increments to ensure a smooth procedure. Start the animal at 2–3% and increase or decrease the delivery of gas based on the animal's status. Maintenance levels for halothane and isoflurane are typically between 1.5–3.0%, but will vary from patient to patient. Anesthetic recovery for animals placed under general anesthesia (alone) is typically within 10–20 minutes after the discontinuation of the gas.

Monitoring of the reptile or amphibian during an anesthetic and/or surgical procedure is often performed by the veterinary technician. The respiratory rate can usually be monitored by direct visualization of the body wall in snakes and lizards, whereas the gular area and "pumping" action of the legs are used to monitor respirations in chelonians. Auscultation of the heart is very difficult in reptiles. Placement of the stethoscope bell directly on the scales results in an irritating friction-generated sound. Esophageal stethoscopes can be used; however, most reptile and amphibian patients are too small to accommodate these large tubes. Crystal ultrasonic dopplers simplify monitoring the heart rate by producing an audible sound that ensures cardiac function. Pulse oximeters have gained in popularity in veterinary hospitals and provide not only the heart rate, but also arterial oxygen saturation. There are a number of different probes that can be purchased with these systems. In mammals, "C-clip" probes are often used, but in reptiles these probes have limited usefulness because the signal cannot penetrate the scales. The cloacal probes appear to work best for reptiles. Although these devices can simplify the role of the veterinary technician, placement and repositioning may be required during the procedure. The mucous membrane color and hydration status should also be monitored on a reptile and amphibian during a surgical procedure. Amphibians should be kept moist throughout the procedure to prevent desiccation. If there is concern that an animal may experience significant blood loss during a procedure, it should be provided fluids (e.g., intravenous or intraosseus).

Reptiles should be provided heat during a surgical procedure. Water-circulating heat pads provide good results and are unlikely to cause thermal burns. When working with these heating elements, it is important to recognize that a reptile's sharp claw could tear the heating pad, so protection (e.g., a towel) should be used. Reptiles are dependent on the environmental temperature to maintain their metabolism and ability to process anesthetics and recover from surgery. Maintaining a reptile at an inappropriate temperature will prolong the recovery, with recovery times lasting 1–3 days in some cases.

Amphibians do not tolerate excessive heat. When performing a procedure on an amphibian it should be done at an appropriate temperature for that animal, typically 76–78°F for tropical species and 74–76°F for temperate species. Attempts to set the ambient room temperature to an appropriate level is preferred over using heat lamps or heating pads, which may overheat the animal and promote desiccation.

Reptiles have very unique respiratory systems. The lungs of the reptile are much simpler than mammals or birds, and reptiles lack a true diaphragm. These anatomical features are important to consider when anesthetizing and maintaining a reptile on inhalant anesthetics. Reptiles normally breathe by movement of their body wall (intercostal muscles), limbs, and viscera. When reptiles or amphibians are under general anesthesia, they may not be capable of breathing on their own and must be ventilated using positive pressure. Typically, 4–5 breaths a minute will be satisfactory. When a reptile or amphibian is ventilated, it is important to use a pressure less than 12 cm of water to prevent their simple sac-like lungs from rupturing.[8]

The veterinary technician plays a vital role in the surgery and is often responsible for managing a number of tasks, including pre-surgical preparation of surgical supplies, preparing an aseptic surgical site, assistance during the surgical procedure, and anesthetic monitoring.

Preparing the surgical suite for a reptile or amphibians patient should follow basic mammalian techniques. The surgical packs should be sterilized using appropriate techniques.

Selection of the appropriate suture material will reduce the possibility of incision dehiscence and poor healing. The absorbable synthetic sutures can be used for ligation and suture placement internally and nylon sutures can be used to close skin incisions. Chromic catgut and stainless steel should not be used in reptiles or amphibians. In reptiles, the skin is considered the primary closing layer because it is unlikely to tear, whereas in mammals the linea alba is the primary closing layer. Skin sutures should remain in a reptile or amphibian patient for 4–6 weeks. This prolonged healing time is associated with the slower metabolism common to ectotherms.

The veterinary technician serves a primary role in monitoring asepsis during the surgical procedure. The surgical suite can become very busy, and it is important that the technician observe that no individual compromises the sterility of the procedure. Preparation of the surgical site should follow standard protocol, wiping from the center of the surgical site in a circular motion until a desired area is sterilized. Preparing the skin of reptiles can be difficult because of the scales, but attempts should be made to remove heavy debris. The skin of an amphibian is very thin, so minimal pressure should be applied when preparing the site. The surgical site should be prepared with a non-irritating solution, such as dilute chlorhexidine (Nolvasan, Fort Dodge Laboratories, Ft. Dodge, IA), followed by isotonic sterile saline. **Alcohol should never be used to disinfect a surgical site on a reptile or amphibian because it creates an evaporative surface that can lead to significant body heat loss.**

During a surgical procedure, the veterinary technician is often expected to manage hemostasis. Hemostasis is essential in the reptile and amphibian patient because any excess loss could prove to be life-threatening. In most cases, simply applying direct pressure using a sponge is sufficient. Do not wipe or smear the blood vessel because it may cause an irritation or further damage the blood vessel. If direct pressure (30–120 seconds) is insufficient to stop the hemorrhage, the veterinary surgeon should consider other techniques such as suture or electrocautery.

Incision irrigation and lavage are other important functions that the veterinary technician performs when assisting the veterinarian during the surgical procedure. The irrigating or lavage fluid should be isotonic (e.g., normal saline) and pre-warmed to the animal's body temperature (37°C is sufficient) to prevent cold stress. Cold stress can rapidly result in a cascade of physiologic changes that can alter the animal's response to the anesthesia. Incisions should be irrigated liberally to improve the veterinary surgeon's visualization of the surgical site. When performing a lavage in the coelomic cavity of the reptile or amphibian, it is important to remember that they lack a diaphragm and that excess irrigation fluid can place excess pressure on the animal's lung(s), making it difficult to breathe. To prevent this problem, lavage limited amounts of fluid at a time, removing any excess with sterile gauze or suction. Be careful when using suction because tissues can be damaged if they are pulled into the suction tube.

After the surgical procedure is completed, the animal should be moved to a clean, warm, quiet area to recover. Remove the animal from the anesthetic machine and allow it to recover on room air. Reptiles are stimulated to breathe when their blood oxygen levels decrease to a threshold; maintaining them on oxygen will only prolong the recovery.[10] The animal should not be extubated until it has started to swallow. Animals that have had a coeliotomy or fracture repair should not be provided climbing branches until the veterinary surgeon feels that the animal is not in danger of wound dehiscence.

DISEASES

The majority of the diseases encountered in pet reptile and amphibian medicine are directly related to inappropriate husbandry. Animals maintained under inappropriate temperatures, provided inadequate diets and housing conditions, are at an increased risk of developing disease.

HUSBANDRY-RELATED PROBLEMS

Thermal Burns

Reptiles will often seek heat to maintain their core body temperature. If an animal is placed in an enclosure that has an exposed light bulb, heating pad, or heat rock as its only source of heat, the animal may remain on the device and develop severe life-threatening burns (Figure 2-14). These cases should be considered emergencies and treated appropriately. In severe burn cases, an animal can lose significant amounts of fluids through the burn sites and should be provided supplemental fluids. The wound should be assessed for severity. Deep contaminated wounds have a guarded prognosis. Prior to initiating wound management, a bacteriological sample should be collected and submitted for a culture and sensitivity to identify potential pathogenic or-

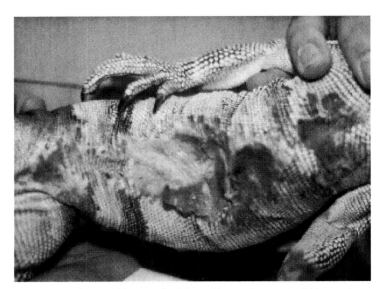

Figure 2-14 Iguana with generalized thermal burns. Owners should be sure to provide alternate sources of heat in order to prevent life-threatening burns such as the ones shown here.

ganisms and an appropriate antibiotic. Wound management should follow standard mammalian protocols. The wound should be irrigated with an isotonic saline solution and a non-irritating cleansing solution, such as chlorhexidine. Topical anti-microbials may be applied to prevent wound contamination. Topical creams or ointments should be applied in a thin coat over the wound, as excessive application can result in anaerobic conditions. Silvadene cream (Par Pharmaceuticals, Inc., Spring Valley, NY) is an excellent anti-microbial cream that can be applied to thermal injuries. Application of a wet-to-dry bandage can be used to reduce wound contamination and encourage wound healing. The bandage should be changed daily until the wound begins to "dry," and then as needed until the granulation tissue is considered adequate. It is important to remember that bandages that include the body wall should not be too restrictive and impede respiration. Animals with severe burns should be placed on antimicrobials. Enrofloxacin (5–10 mg/kg PO SID) or trimethoprim-sulfa (15 mg/kg PO SID) provide excellent coverage and can be initiated while sensitivity is pending.

Prey Bites

Reptiles and amphibians only hunt food when they are hungry. Most owners offer their reptiles and amphibians live-foods assuming that the pet will eat, or at least kill, the food item. Unfortunately, this is not always the case. Many prey items, including rodents and insects, will "attack" the predator if left unattended (Figure 2-15). There are a number of reports citing large snakes that died from wounds inflicted by a mouse or rat. Even common crickets have been observed to "feed" on juvenile lizards. A prey bite should always be managed as a contaminated wound. (See thermal burns.) Owners should be educated as to the dangers of feeding live prey and directed to observe their pet during feedings. All mammalian prey items (e.g., rats and mice) should be humanely euthanized before being fed to reptiles.

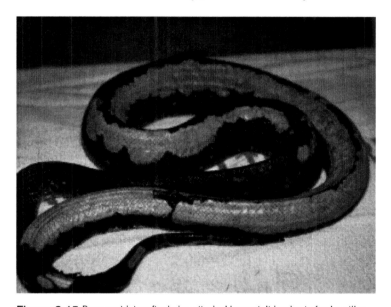

Figure 2-15 Boa constrictor after being attacked by a rat. It is wise to feed reptiles only killed food in order to avoid serious prey bites.

Dysecdysis

Reptiles shed the outer epidermal layer of their skin as they grow. In juvenile animals, shedding (ecdysis) occurs regularly and slows as the animal matures. Shedding of the skin is a routine and necessary behavior that all reptiles experience; however, patterns of shedding differ between species. Chelonians and lizards routinely shed their skin in pieces, whereas snakes shed their skin in one entire piece. Most of the problems associated with shedding (dysecdysis) are reported in snakes, although dysecdysis can occur in all reptiles. Causes of dysecdysis in reptiles have been associated with low environmental humidity and temperature, ectoparasites, traumatic wounds, systemic disease, mishandling, and the lack of an adequate surface to assist with shedding. Treatment for dysecdysis should include correcting any environmental and medical problems and soaking the animal in a shallow, warm (82–84°F) water bath. The depth of the water bath should not exceed 1/2 of the height of the animal. Never use a human water receptacle (e.g., bathtub or sink) to soak a reptile. After soaking, a soft, cotton towel can be used to gently wipe the animal down and remove any excess shed. Do not pull at skin that is not ready to come off because you can damage the underlying skin. Owners should be made aware of the importance of checking the spectacles or eye caps to make sure that they are removed after every shed. Retained spectacles can develop into sub-spectacular abscesses, which can lead to the loss of the eye if not managed appropriately.

NUTRITIONAL DISEASES

Secondary Nutritional Hyperparathyroidism

The most common nutritional disease reported in reptiles is secondary nutritional hyperparathyroidism (SNH). SNH may occur as a result of a calcium deficient diet, phosphorus rich diet, and/or vitamin D$_3$ deficiency. In this disease process, the parathyroid glands are activated and release parathormone, which mobilizes calcium from the skeleton for the animal to meet its daily needs. A thorough history will often guide a veterinarian in the diagnosis of this disease. Animals suffering from SNH are often young,

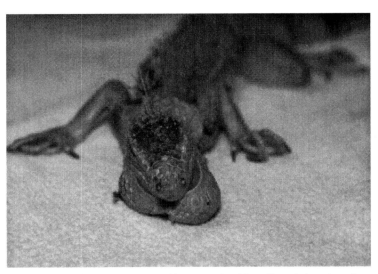

Figure 2-16A Secondary nutritional hyperparathyroidism. Frontal view of swollen mandibles (fibrous osteodystrophy).

fast-growing animals or adult reproductively active females maintained at an inappropriate ETR (reduced metabolism), offered a calcium deficient diet, excessive phosphorus diet, and/or not exposed to ultraviolet B wavelength light (synthesis of vitamin D_3). On physical examination, the animal often has muscle tremors and fasciculations, "swollen" mandibles (Figures 2-16A and 2-16B) and long bones (fibrous osteodystrophy), and may suffer from seizures. Clinical diagnosis is made from a thorough history, physical examination, and radiographs. These animals should be considered critical care cases, and therapy should be initiated immedi-

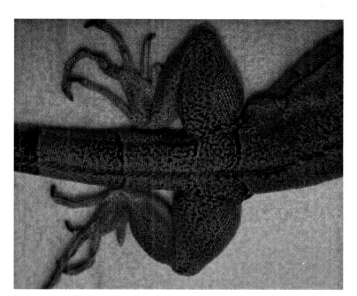

Figure 2-16B Rear view of an iguana with secondary nutritional hyperparathyroidism.

ately. Medical management includes supplemental calcium and vitamin D therapy, fluids to rehydrate animals, enteral support to maintain energy demands, and treatment of secondary problems, such as splinting pathologic fractures.

Hypovitaminosis A

Chelonians offered inappropriate diets often develop hypovitaminosis A. Animals presenting with hypovitaminosis A are often young, fast-growing animals or long-term wild caught specimens maintained at inappropriate temperatures and offered a restricted, vitamin A deficient diet. On physical examination, the animals will often have unilateral or bilateral blepharoedema (swelling of the eyelids), a nasal and ocular discharge, diarrhea, pneumonia, aural abscesses, and hyperkeratosis. Vitamin A deficiency leads to changes in the epithelial lining of the respiratory tract, oral cavity, skin, and urinary tract. The resulting squamous metaplasia reduces the tight junctions formed by the cells and allows for opportunistic pathogens to invade.[11] Diagnosis is often made from the history, physical examination, and response to treatment. Animals with respiratory disease should have a culture and sensitivity performed to evaluate appropriate antimicrobial therapy to manage opportunistic infections. Animals considered to have hypovitaminosis A should be administered vitamin A (500–1,500 IU/kg every 10 days for 1–4 treatments).[12] Over-supplementation of vitamin A can lead to iatrogenic hypervitaminosis A. Hypervitaminosis A leads to skin sloughing and can be life-threatening.

Gout

Gout results from the deposition of monosodium urate crystals into the viscera (visceral gout) or joints (articular gout) as a result of the body synthesizing too much uric acid (e.g., high protein diets), dehydration, or renal impairment. Animals presenting with gout are often adult animals and may be herbivores, omnivores, or carnivores. Generally, these animals are reported to be in good health, but become acutely depressed and lethargic. A review of husbandry practices will often reveal that these animals have been offered an inappropriate diet or not provided sufficient access to a water source. On physical examination, these animals are clinically dehydrated, have poor muscling condition, and are in overall poor condition. A thorough history, physical examination, plasma chemistry profile, and radiographs will help establish a diagnosis. Reptiles and amphibians with gout often have a hyperuricemia; however, animals with gout can have normal plasma uric acid levels. If the kidneys are impaired as a result of the monosodium urate crystallization, the calcium:phosphorus levels will most likely be inverse (<1:1). Radiograph of a reptile with gout may reveal lesions in joints or viscera. The goal of treatment for a reptile or amphibian with gout is to correct the original dietary (e.g., reduce dietary proteins, offer correct diet) and environmental (e.g., ad libitum access to water) problems, reduce uric acid production in the body (Allopurinol, 20 mg/kg PO SID), and increase urate excretion (Probenecid, 250 mg/kg, PO SID).[13] The prognosis for these cases is guarded.

INFECTIOUS DISEASES

Reptiles and amphibians are susceptible to a number of infectious agents, including viruses, bacteria, and fungi. The majority of cases presented to veterinary hospitals are directly related to inappropriate management. When a reptile or amphibian is maintained at low environmental temperatures, its immune function is reduced and it is prone to opportunistic infections. Another source of infectious diseases for reptile collections is inadequate quarantine. Newly acquired animals should be segregated from other reptiles to ensure that they are not shedding infectious agents that might contaminate a collection. The quarantine period for a reptile or amphibian should be a minimum of 60–90 days.[14]

ABSCESSES

Abscesses are a common finding in animals that are managed under inappropriate conditions. Abscesses are often the result of an infectious origin (e.g., bacterial infection), foreign body, or parasite. Abscesses in reptiles and amphibians can be found anywhere on the body and are commonly located on the toes and tail and in the oral cavity (Figure 2-17). Abscesses are often firm, well-circumscribed lesions. Diagnosis of an abscess is often made from the history, physical examination and the results of an aspirate or biopsy of the mass. Reptile abscesses are typically caseous or "cheesy" in nature, rather than liquefactive or "pus" as in mammals. This difference is related to the reduced enzymatic fire-power that reptile cells possess in relation to higher vertebrates. Successful management of an abscess in a reptile or amphibian requires incision and curettage. Simply initiating systemic antibiotic therapy will be insufficient because the inciting cause or nidus, if bacterial, is often located in the center of the abscess and will be unaffected by any drugs. A local anesthetic line, or ring block using lidocaine, should be performed prior to making the incision. A microbiological sample should be collected for culture and sensitivity once the incision is made. Caseous abscesses can generally be scooped out of the incision. The open wound should then be irrigated with a non-irritating disinfectant, such as diluted

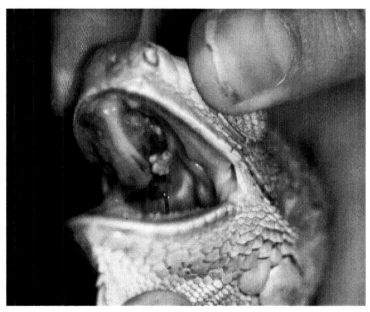

Figure 2-17 An iguana with an oral abscess.

chlorhexidine. A single, localized abscess can often be managed by irrigating it and applying a topical antimicrobial ointment. Generalized abscesses require systemic treatment and a systemic antibiotic, based on the sensitivity findings.

VIRUSES

As diagnostic techniques to identify viruses improve, more and more of these pathogens are being associated with disease in reptiles and amphibians. The viruses that have received the most attention in pet reptile medicine are the paramyxovirus and retrovirus.

Paramyxoviruses are primarily associated with viperid snakes, although they have also been identified in nonviperid snakes.[19, 20] This virus is typically spread from contact with respiratory secretions. Affected animals display clinical signs associated with respiratory disease, such as nasal and oral discharge, open-mouth breathing, increased lung sounds, and possible neurologic signs, including tremors and seizures. Diagnosis can be made antemortem from a blood test or postmortem from a histologic diagnosis.[21] There is no effective treatment for this virus.

Inclusion body disease is associated with a retrovirus that primarily affects snakes in the family Boidae (e.g., boas and pythons). The method of transmission of this virus is unknown, but it is suspected that snake mites (*Ophionyssus natricis*) may play a role. Affected boa constrictors present with chronic regurgitation, but may develop neurologic signs, including loss of righting reflex, tremors, and disorientation, as the disease progresses. Affected pythons develop severe neurologic signs, similar to that described for the boas, which progressively worsen. Animals typically succumb to this disease as a result of secondary infections and starvation. Diagnosis can be made antemortem from surgical biopsies and postmortem from histopathologic examination. There is no effective treatment for this virus. Affected animals should be euthanized to prevent the spread of the virus to other snakes.

Adenovirus and dependovirus may cause significant mortalities in captive raised lizards (e.g., bearded dragons) and snakes (e.g., kingsnakes). Affected animals present for anorexia, regurgitation, muscle wasting, and death. The exact method of transmission of this virus is not well known, but it is most commonly reported when large numbers of juvenile animals are housed together. It has been suggested that unaffected adult animals may serve as a source of the virus for hatchling reptiles. Diagnosis of this virus is routinely made at necropsy. Unfortunately, there is no effective treatment for this virus at this time.

ZOONOTIC DISEASES

The veterinarian and veterinary technician serve vital roles in educating their support staff and clients about the potential diseases that their patients (reptiles and amphibians) may spread to humans (zoonoses). Many zoonotic diseases can be prevented by practicing strict hygiene and using common sense. Exotic pet animals should not be recommended for households with infants and young children, immunocompromised individuals, or the elderly because the immune systems in these groups of individuals are often naive or inefficient at protecting them against most pathogens.

The most notorious reptile zoonosis is salmonellosis. *Salmonella* spp. is a Gram-negative rod that is a facultative anaerobe. There are more than 2,435 serotypes of *Salmonella* spp.[18] All *Salmonella* spp. should be considered pathogenic to humans.

In the early 1970s, there were over 280,000 human cases of Salmonellosis in the United States directly attributed to reptiles (turtles).[19] Attempts to certify the animals as *Salmonella* spp. free in the United States failed because the animals were found to be latent shedders of the organism, i.e., they could test negative one week and positive weeks or months later. In 1975, the United States Food and Drug Administration put an interstate shipping ban on turtles with a carapace under 4 inches, effectively halting the sale of turtles in the United States. The ban on turtles proved to be successful as follow-up research indicated that a 77% decrease in turtle-associated Salmonellosis.[20]

During the late 1980s and 1990s reptile-associated Salmonellosis has again received national attention. There have been a number of reported cases where infants have been hospitalized, with one infant dying, after exposure to green iguanas or other pet reptiles. These cases differed from the turtle-associated Salmonellosis cases because the infants did not have direct contact with the animal. Owners should be warned of these potential hazards; and it should be suggested that households with infants, elderly, or immunocompromised individuals not keep these animals as pets. Otherwise, owners should practice strict hygiene practices such as washing their hands, cleaning fecal wastes with an appropriate disinfectant, and wearing gloves during the procedure. They should also not handle the animals near human food preparation sites or wash receptacles (e.g., sinks and bathtubs) and not allow the animal free roam within a human domicile.

There are other species of bacteria (Gram-positive and Gram-negative) that have been isolated from clinically healthy and diseased reptiles that can cause disease in humans, including: *Aeromonas* spp., *Campylobacter* spp., *Citrobacter* spp., *Edwardsiella* spp., *Escherichia coli*, *Klebsiella* spp., *Mycobacterium* spp., *Pasteurella* spp., *Proteus* spp., *Staphylococcus* spp., and *Streptococcus* spp. The population at risk is similar to that defined for Salmonellosis and includes infants, immunocompromised individuals, and the elderly—although clinically healthy adults may develop infections under certain circumstances. Humans may be exposed to these pathogens through wound contamination (e.g., scratch or bite wounds), water exposure, or fecal-oral exposure. Adhering to strict hygiene practices, such as hand washing, wearing protective gloves when cleaning reptile enclosures, and not handling or allowing the animals near human food preparation sites should prevent disease.

REFERENCES

1. Frye, F.L. and Boyer, T.H. "Captive Reptile Husbandry." In Frye, F.L., ed. *Reptile Care.* Neptune City: Tropical Fish Hobbyists Publications, Inc., 1991: 23–26.

2. Allen, M.E., Oftedal, O.T., and Ullrey, E.D. "Effect of Dietary Calcium Concentration on Mineral Composition in Fox Geckos (*Hemidactylus garnoti*) and Cuban Tree Frogs (*Osteopilus septentrionalis*)," *Journal of Zoo and Wildlife Medicine* 24 (1993): 118.

3. Donoghue, S. and Langenberg, J. "Nutrition." In Mader, D.R. ed., *Reptile Medicine and Surgery*. Philadelphia: W.B. Saunders, 1996: 148–174.

4. Boyer, T.H. "Metabolic Bone Disease." In Mader, D.R. ed., *Reptile Medicine and Surgery*. Philadelphia: W.B. Saunders, 1996: 385–392.

5. Jacobsen, E.R. "Blood Collection Techniques in Reptiles: Laboratory Investigations." In Fowler, M.E. ed., *Zoo and Wild Animal Medicine: Current Therapy 3*. Philadelphia: W.B. Saunders, 1993: 144–52

6. Wright, K.M. "Amphibian Husbandry and Medicine." In Mader, D.R. ed., *Reptile Medicine and Surgery*. Philadelphia: W.B. Saunders, 1996: 436–459.

7. Lane, T.J. and Mader, D.R. "Parasitology." In Mader, D.R. ed., *Reptile Medicine and Surgery*. Philadelphia: W.B. Saunders, 1996: 185–203.

8. Bennet, R.A. "Anesthesia." In Mader, D.R. ed., *Reptile Medicine and Surgery*. Philadelphia: W.B. Saunders, 1996: 241–247.

9. Divers, S.J. "The Use of Propofol in Reptile Anesthesia." Proceedings of the Association of Reptile and Amphibian Veterinarians, 1996: 57–59.

10. Diethelm, G. and Mader, D.R. "The Effect of FlO$_2$ on Post Anesthetic Recovery Times in the Green Iguana," Proceedings of the Association of Reptile and Amphibian Veterinarians, 1999: 169–170.

11. Frye, F.L. "Nutritional Disorders in Reptiles." In Hoff, G.L., Frye, F.L., and Jacobson, E.R. ed., *Diseases of Amphibians and Reptiles*. New York: Plenum Press, 1984: 640–642.

12. Fowler, M.E. "Comparison of Respiratory Infection and Hypovitaminosis A in a Desert Tortoise." In Montali, R.J. and Migaki, G. eds., *Comparative Pathology of Zoo Animals*. Washington, D.C., Smithsonian Institute, 1980: 93–97.

13. Mader, D.R. "Gout." In Mader D.R. ed., *Reptile Medicine and Surgery*. Philadelphia: W.B. Saunders, 1996: 374–379.

14. Lloyd, M.L., Flanagan, J.P. "Recent Developments in Ophidian Paramyxovirus Research and Recommendations on Control. South Padre Island, Texas," Proceedings of the American Association of Zoo Veterinarians, 1990: 151–6.

15. Ahne, W., Neubert W.J., and Thomson, I. "Reptilian Viruses: Isolation of Myxovirus-like Particles from the Snake *Elaphe oxycephala*." *Journal of American Veterinary Medicine* 34 (1987): 607.

16. Jacobsen, E.R., Gaskin, J.M., Simpson, C. et al., "Paramyxo-like Virus Infection in a Rock Rattlesnake," *Journal of American Veterinary Medicine*, 177 (9): 796, 1980.

17. Schumacher, J. "Viral Diseases." In Mader, D.R. ed., *Reptile Medicine and Surgery*. Philadelphia: W.B. Saunders, 1996: 224–234.

18. Popoff, M.Y. and Leminor, L. "Antigenic Formulas of the *Salmonella* Serovars," 7th revision. World Health Organization Collaborating Center for Reference Research on *Salmonella*, Pasteur Institute, Paris, France, 1997.

19. Lamm S.H., Taylor, A., Gangarosa, E.J. et al., "Turtle-Associated Salmonellosis I: An Estimation of the Magnitude of the Problem in the United States, 1970–1971," *American Journal of Epidemiology*, 95 (6): 511–517, 1972.

20. Cohen, M.L., Potter, M., Pollard et al., "Turtle-Associated Salmonellosis in the United States. Effect of Public Health Action, 1970–1976," *Journal of the American Veterinary Medical Association* 12, no. 243, 1980: 1247–1249.

21. Jacobson, E.R. "Use of Chemotherapeutics in Reptile Medicine." In Jacobson, E.R. and Kollias, G.V. eds., *Exotic Animals*. New York: Churchill Livingston, 1988: 35–48.

22. Jacobson, E.R. "Antimicrobial Drug Use in Reptiles." In Prescott, J.F. and Baggot, J.D. eds., *Antimicrobial Therapy in Veterinary Medicine*. Ames, Iowa: Iowa State University Press, 1993: 543–552.

23. Allen, D.G., Pringle, J.K., and Smith, D. *Handbook of Veterinary Drugs*. Philadelphia: J.B. Lippincott, 1993: 534–567.

24. Klingenberg, R.J. "Therapeutic." In Mader, D.R. ed., *Reptile Medicine and Surgery*. Philadelphia: W.B. Saunders, 1996: 299–321.

25. Jacobson, E.R. "Snakes." *Veterinary Clinics of North America Small Animal Practice* 23 (1993) 1179–1212.

CHAPTER 3

FERRETS

INTRODUCTION

The ferret, *Mustela putorius furo*, belongs to the order Carnivora and the family Mustelidae. These animals continue to gain in popularity as a pet with over 7 million animals in the United States.[1] The ferret has endeared itself to humans because of its "spunky" personality and small stature. The ferret has also become quite popular in urban domiciles (e.g., apartments) that might be too small to house dogs or cats.

Domestication of the ferret is not recent, since it has been recorded that ferrets were used for hunting over 2,000 years ago.[2] The ferret was originally introduced into the United States over 300 years ago.[3] In other parts of the world, such as England, the ferret serves in a working role as a hunter of rabbits and rodents. The ferret is also used extensively in research.

Although the domestic ferret continues to gain in popularity in the United States, it cannot legally be kept as a pet in all states. The ferret has developed an unfortunate reputation in certain areas as being considered dangerous around children or a threat to native wildlife. Local ordinances in certain "ferret-legal" states may prohibit ferrets as pets, so it is important to research the laws in your state and local municipality to protect yourself and your clients. In many states, the wildlife and fisheries department regulates permits for domestic ferrets; it should be contacted regarding official regulations.

Success in working with the ferret, as with all exotic species, requires veterinary technicians to develop a basic knowledge of the anatomy and physiology of the animal (Table 3-1), so that they can perform a thorough physical examination, administer medical therapy, and answer an owner's questions about his pet.

Table 3-1
Ferret Basic Information

Body weight	Adult male (Hob)	
	Intact	1.0–2.0 kg[3]
	Neutered	0.7–1.1 kg
	Adult female (Jill)	
	Intact	0.5–1.0 kg[3]
	Neutered	0.5–0.7 kg
	Birth weight (Kit)	8–10 grams[3]
Temperature, pulse and respiration	Rectal body temperature	100–103°F
	Normal heart rate	170–230 beats/minute
	Normal respiratory rate	25–40 breaths/minute
Reproductive cycle	Sexual maturity	4–8 months of age[3]
	Gestation	41–42 days[3]
	Estrous cycle	Induced ovulator
	Weaning age	6–8 weeks
	Life span	4–9 years average up to 11–12 years

ANATOMY

The technician should become familiar with those anatomical characteristics in the ferret that differ from other domestic mammals. The ferret has a long tubular body that enables it to maneuver through burrows when hunting prey. The ferret has sharp, nonretractable claws. Ferrets use these to dig and burrow, and ferret owners are often scratched by their pets while playing with them. Ferret owners may request to have their pet declawed; however, the procedure would be very painful and should never be performed. The majority of ferrets offered for sale in pet shops are descented and neutered. Neutered animals may weigh significantly less than their intact counterparts (Table 3-1). Ferrets may lose a significant amount of weight during the summer months, only to gain the weight back in the winter. Indoor domestic ferrets may experience a 10–30% weight change, whereas an outdoor intact animal may fluctuate by as much as 40% of its body weight.[3] There are over 30 hair coat color variations recognized in the domestic ferret. The most common colors, sable and albino, are naturally occurring patterns, while many of the other variations are the result of selective breeding (Figures 3-1 and 3-2). Ferrets

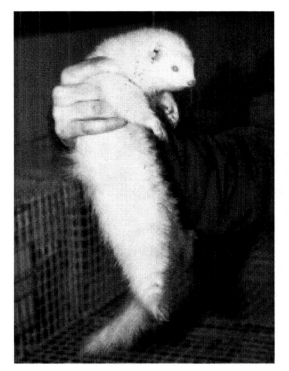

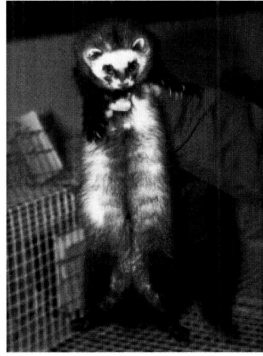

Figure 3-1 Albino ferret. The distinguishing characteristics of an albino ferret are its white coat and pink eyes.

Figure 3-2 A sable ferret is identified by distinctive black markings on his face and body.

undergo routine spring and fall seasonal molts, similar to domestic dogs. Ferrets have very thick skin and a technician may find it difficult to inject vaccinations between the shoulders. The ferret has a pair of anal glands that produce a musky odor. Commercial breeding farms descent and neuter kits prior to shipping them to pet stores, while private breeders will often leave that option to the new owner. Female ferrets are induced ovulators and must be bred by a male to stimulate ovulation. A female that is not bred or spayed may develop a life-threatening estrogen induced anemia. Male ferrets have a j-shaped os penis. The ferret is a true carnivore and has a relatively short gastrointestinal tract. Ferrets are capable of processing a meal within 3–4 hours.

HUSBANDRY

ENVIRONMENTAL CONCERNS

Ferrets may be maintained indoors or outdoors. They are primarily maintained indoors in the United States, whereas they are often maintained outdoors in Europe. Ferrets kept outdoors should be protected from extremes of heat and cold. During the summer months, animals should be provided shelter and fresh water and should be removed from the direct sun. Ferrets do not tolerate temperatures over 88–90°F. In the winter, animals should be provided a shelter with straw or hay. When the temperature drops below freezing (32°F), the ferrets should be brought into a warm shelter.

Ferrets should be provided a well-ventilated, spacious enclosure. Glass fish tanks are not suitable for ferrets because they do not allow for adequate ventilation. Animals maintained in glass enclosures often develop respiratory problems. Galvanized metal cages or wood-frame cages are routinely used to house ferrets. Galvanized metal is composed of zinc and may predispose those that lick and chew the bars to heavy metal toxicity. Reports of heavy metal toxicity in ferrets are rare, but should be considered in animals that display neurologic signs.

The enclosure should be large enough to provide the animal an area to sleep, eat, exercise, and have a latrine. Ferrets urinate and defecate in corners and can be trained to use a litter-box. Owners may need to place a litter-box in multiple corners to ensure their pet will use it. Litter pans should have low sides to allow the animals easy access. Fecal and urine material should be removed from the litter pan daily.

Ferrets naturally tend to burrow and hide when they sleep, and owners should provide their pet with a sleeping shelter. There are a number of commercial ferret hammocks or slings that can be provided, although most old towels or shirts work fine. Owners should observe their pet closely to ensure that it does not attempt to ingest any of the material. Cardboard box shelter may be provided to animals that are at risk with the cloth material.

Ferrets should remain in their cage and only be allowed to roam free in a home under close supervision. These animals are capable of fitting into small crevices between furniture and ventilation systems and are notorious for getting into trouble. The ingestion of foreign material is the most common problem reported in unsupervised ferrets. Commercial ferret harnesses may be used to walk an animal indoors or outdoors.

NUTRITION

Ferrets are true carnivores, as evidenced by their relatively short gastrointestinal tract. The gastrointestinal transit time of the ferret is rapid (3–4 hours), so food quality is important to ensure maximal nutritional benefit. The diet of a ferret should consist primarily of high quality protein and fat. The exact nutritional requirements for the ferret have not been established, although it is generally accepted that adult altered animals require 30–40% protein and 18–20% fat.[5] Breeding animals and young, fast-growing kits require significantly more protein (minimum 35%) and fat (minimum 25%). Although readily accepted by ferrets, carbohydrates (e.g., sweets) should be minimized in the animal's diet. The short gastrointestinal tract of the ferret is not dependent on dietary fiber, as is the case in herbivores. Most commercial ferret diets contain minimal quantities of fiber.

There are a number of commercial diets that may provide a ferret with adequate nutrition. In recent years, commercial ferret diets have been offered for sale at the retail pet store. Ferret owners should read the labels of commercial diets to ensure that the appropriate levels of protein and fat are offered, based on the animal's age and reproductive status. Commercial feline growth diets are also routinely recommended for ferrets. Again, the ingredient list should be evaluated and recommendations made based on the animal's needs. Canine diets should never be recommended for ferrets because they do not provide adequate protein or fat and contain significant amount of carbohydrates. A ferret may be offered food *ad lib*. Ferret diets may be supplemented with lean meats such as chicken or beef, or meat-base (onion salt-free) baby foods.

Ferrets should be offered fresh, clean water daily. Water may be offered in heavy ceramic water bowls or hanging sipper bottles. The bowl should be placed in a corner where it is unlikely a ferret can tip it over. Water sipper bottles should be placed in an area of the cage that is readily accessible to the animal. Water-soluble vitamins are not necessary for ferrets that are provided a good quality commercial ferret or feline growth diet.

GROOMING

Ferrets naturally have a musky odor, which is especially evident in intact animals during the breeding season. Ferrets do not require regular bathing; however, they may be bathed once a month, if desired. The most appropriate shampoo is one that is pH balanced, such as a commercial ferret or kitten shampoo. Excessive bathing may lead to the development of dry, pruritic skin.

In the wild, ferrets utilize their sharp nails to dig. In captivity this may be annoying and painful. Ferret nails may be trimmed in the same fashion described for dogs and cats. If the nail is cut short and the animal bleeds, an appropriate styptic powder may be applied. On occasion, we are asked about the possibility of declawing a ferret. Ferret nails are nonretractable, like a dog's nails. An onchiectomy should never be performed on this species.

Ferrets may develop significant dental tartar over time. To prevent potential dental problems, the animal's teeth should be brushed regularly. The commercially available toothbrushes and toothpaste available for use in dogs and cats may also be used to clean ferret teeth.

HISTORY

A thorough history is essential to making an appropriate diagnosis for any exotic animal case because many of the problems identified in exotic animals are directly related to inappropriate husbandry (Figure 3-3). A veterinary technician should first

Ferret History Form	Date:		
RDVM info	Admitting Clinician:		
	Appt. Time:		

| Name of Ferret:_____ | Color variety:_____ | Sex:_____ | Age:____ |

Background Information:
Length of time owned:_____   Where acquired? Breeder ❏ Pet Store ❏ Other_____
Vaccination History: Distemper_____   Rabies_____
                 Date of Vaccination   Date of Vaccination
On Heartworm preventative? Yes ❏ No ❏   Has ferret been tested for heartworms?_____
How often is ferret handled? Daily ❏ Occasionally ❏ Never ❏   Character of Feces_____

Husbandry:
Housed Indoors/Outdoors?_____   Is ferret allowed to roam free in the house? Yes ❏ No ❏
Where is cage located?_____ Size of Cage_____
Type of Caging:_____   Galvanized? Yes ❏   No ❏

Cage Substrate?_____ How often is caged cleaned?_____
Is there a Litter Pan present in cage?_____ What brand of litter is used in pan?_____
What type of disinfectant is used when cleaning cage?_____
Types of furniture within cage?_____
Types of toys_____
Nutrition:
<u>Type of food offered:</u>
–Cat Food? No ❏ Yes ❏   If yes, what brand?_____ Amount fed/frequency:_____

–Ferret Food? No ❏ Yes ❏   If yes, what type?_____ Amount fed/frequency:_____

--Supplement/Treats offered and frequency?_____

Water source?_____ How often is water changed?_____

Any other pets? No ❏ Yes ❏ If yes, specify_____ Do other pets interact with ferret? Y/N

Any other ferrets? No ❏ Yes ❏ Specify_____
Are ferrets housed together or singly?_____ If not housed together, do the ferrets interact?_____
Any new additions to the ferret population? No ❏ Yes ❏ If yes, specify_____

Past Medical History/Problems:

Current Presenting Problem:

Duration of Complaint:

Figure 3-3 An example of a typical history form that can be used to evaluate a ferret's health.

Table 3-2
Ferret Hematologic Reference Ranges[4,6]

	Albino		Fitch	
	Male	**Female**	**Male**	**Female**
PCV (%)	55 (44–61)	49 (42–55)	43 (36-50)	48 (47-51)
RBC ($10^6/\mu l$)	10.2 (7.3–12.2)	8.1 (6.8–9.8)	———	———
Hemoglobin (g/dl)	17.8 (16.3–18.2)	16.2 (14.8–17.4)	14.3 (12.0–16.3)	15.9 (15.2–17.4)
Leukocytes ($10^3/\mu l$)	9.7 (4.4–19.1)	10.5 (4.0–18.2)	11.3 (7.7–15.4)	5.9 (2.5–8.6)
Neutrophils (%)	57 (11–82)	59.5 (43–84)	40.1 (24–78)	31.1 (12–41)
Bands (%)	———	———	0.9 (0–2.2)	1.7 (0–4.2)
Lymphocytes (%)	35.6 (12–54)	33.4 (12–50)	49.7 (28–69)	58 (25–95)
Eosinophils (%)	2.4 (0–7)	2.6 (0–5)	2.3 (0–7)	3.6 (1–9)
Monocytes (%)	4.4 (0–9)	4.4 (2–8)	6.6 (3.4–8.2)	4.5 (1.7–6.3)
Basophils (%)	0.1 (0–2)	0.2 (0–1)	0.7 (0–2.7)	0.8 (0–2.9)
Platelets ($10^3/\mu l$)	453 (297–730)	545 (310–910)	———	———
Reticuloytes (%)	4.0 (1–12)	5.3 (2–14)	———	———

collect the signalment, including age, breed, sex, and color variety. Knowledge of the animal's age and gender can be useful when developing a differential diagnosis list. For example, an adult intact female ferret with a history of weakness and lethargy may be suffering from an estrogen-induced anemia, whereas an adult male or female kit would be very unlikely to develop the same problem. Knowledge of the color variety is also important because differences in physiologic parameters, such as hematology, can vary. (See Tables 3-2 and 3-3.)

After collecting the signalment, the history should focus on background information, including: where the animal was acquired; length of time owned; if the owner has other pets or ferrets; if he recently acquired another ferret; the interaction between the owner and his pet; and the animal's vaccination (canine distemper virus and rabies) and heartworm preventative status. This information should provide the technician with an initial understanding of the client's knowledge of his pet ferret.

Table 3–3
Ferret Serum Biochemistry Reference Ranges[4,6,7]

	Albino–Hob	Fitch–Hob
Glucose (mg/dl)	136 (94–207)	101 (63–134)
Blood urea nitrogen (mg/dl)	22 (10–45)	28 (12–43)
Creatinine (mg/dl)	0.6 (0.4–0.9)	0.4 (0.2–0.6)
Total bilirubin (mg/dl)	< 1.0	————
Cholesterol (mg/dl)	165 (64–296)	————
Calcium (mg/dl)	9.2 (8.0–11.8)	9.3 (8.6–10.5)
Phosphorus (mg/dl)	5.9 (4.0–9.1)	6.5 (5.6–8.7)
Alkaline phosphatase (IU/L)	23 (9–84)	53 (30–120)
Alanine aminotransferase (IU/L)	————	170 (82–289)
Aspartate aminotransferase (IU/L)	65 (28–120)	————
Sodium (mmol/L)	148 (137–162)	152 (146–160)
Chloride (mmol/L)	116 (106–125)	115 (102–121)
Potassium (mmol/L)	5.9 (4.5–7.7)	4.9 (4.3–5.3)
Total protein (g/dl)	6.0 (5.1–7.4)	5.9 (5.3–7.2)
Albumin (g/dl)	3.2 (2.6–3.8)	3.7 (3.3–4.1)
Globulin (g/dl)	————	1.8 (1.3–2.1)

The next set of questions should focus on how the animal is managed at home (husbandry), including: whether the animal is housed indoors or outdoors; if it has supervised or unsupervised run in the house; cage size and material; cage location in the house; whether ferrets are housed singly or together; substrate used in the cage; how often the cage is cleaned and the type of disinfectant; whether a litter pan is used; the brand of cat litter; and the types of cage furniture (e.g., ferret hammock) and toys. Questions about the animal's nutrition are also important and should include: type of food (e.g., ferret or cat), brand, amount fed, frequency, supplements, water source, and how often the food and water are changed.

Finally, questions should focus on the animal's current health status and should include past medical history, current presenting problem, and the duration of the complaint. Although it is natural to want to focus on the problem at hand, a great deal of information may be lost if the history is not collected in a thorough and systematic approach.

RESTRAINT

Ferrets should be transported in a carrier when they visit the veterinarian. If these animals are allowed free roam in a car during transport, they may get into a particular area that makes them difficult to retrieve, or ingest foreign material (e.g., coins) lying on the floor of the automobile. Ferrets should also be maintained in a transport carrier while they are in the waiting room to prevent contact with other animals and/or a dog or cat attack. To reduce stress during the transport, a towel can be placed in the carrier to provide the animal a place to burrow and hide.

Using the appropriate technique when restraining a ferret is essential to the protection of the veterinarian, the technician, and the animal. Ferrets can be safely restrained by scruffing—a technique commonly used by the jill to move her kits. Scruffing is accomplished by grasping the skin over the dorsal cervical area with the index finger and thumb (Figure 3-4). Once the animal is scruffed, it will often relax and offer little resistance. The handler's second hand should be placed along the spine to protect it from injury. Do not hold the rear legs or allow the animal to place them on the table, as this often stimulates the animal to struggle. Ferrets will often yawn while being scruffed, which will facilitate examination of the oral cavity. Adult pet ferrets rarely bite, but may if they are in pain. A ferret will often make a hissing sound to warn a handler of their dissatisfaction prior to attempting to bite. Animals that are too difficult to handle may be sedated using anesthetics. Kits, on the other hand, are naturally very playful (and teething) and are likely to bite. Moribund

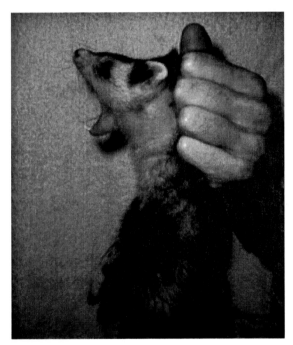

Figure 3-4 "Scruffing" a ferret. Although grabbing a ferret by the nape appears traumatic, it is actually the preferred method of holding a ferret to perform a physical examination.

and cooperative animals may simply be restrained on the examination table; however, any invasive procedure (e.g., vaccination, rectal temperature, injection) will require scruffing.

PHYSICAL EXAMINATION

Ferrets are stoic animals and may not display overt clinical signs until late into the course of the disease; therefore, a thorough physical examination should be performed on every animal presented to the veterinary hospital. Physical examination of the ferret should follow the standard protocol recommended for domestic species.

The ferret should be observed from a distance to assess those functions, such as locomotion, behavior, and respiration, which may be altered by restraint. The ferret should be mobile, aware of its surroundings, and its breathing pattern consistent and not labored. Coughing, sneezing, or nasal discharge should be considered abnormal findings.

When removed from the carrier, the animal should be bright, alert, and responsive. If the ferret is limp or nonresponsive, then the animal should be considered abnormal. Proper restraint is essential to perform a thorough physical examination. The animal's eyes should be clear and free of discharge. A fluorescein stain should be performed on any animal in which a corneal ulcer is suspected. The nares should be clear and free of any crusting or discharge. Ferret ears may have a dark, ceruminous wax build-up. If an excessive amount of wax is identified, a cotton-tip applicator should be dipped in mineral oil and a sample of the wax collected and tested for ear mites (*Otodectes cyonotis*). The oral cavity should be thoroughly evaluated. The teeth should be free of obvious dental caries or fractures. The amount of dental tartar should be recorded, and animals with moderate to severe dental tartar should be scheduled for a tooth cleaning. The mucous membranes should be moist and pink. The capillary refill time should be less than 2 seconds. Hydration status may be assessed by evaluating the mucous membrane quality and capillary refill time, packed cell volume, skin elasticity, and retrobulbar fat. A ferret with a decreased capillary refill time (> 2 seconds) and slowed skin elasticity should be considered 5% dehydrated. When an animal also presents with sunken eyes, resulting from the loss of fluid from the retrobulbar fat, the animal should be considered at least 10–12% dehydrated.

The length and condition of a ferret's hair coat may vary with the season, with the hair coat being much thinner in the summer than during the winter. Seasonal tail alopecia is also a common finding reported in ferrets during the late summer and early fall. Animals that develop symmetrical alopecia and/or thinning of the skin may have an endocrinopathy (e.g., adrenal gland disease) (Figure 3-5). Thoroughly evaluate the skin for defects such as tumors; mast cell tumors are an especially common finding in ferrets. The ferret has peripheral lymph nodes similar to the cat and dog, including the cervical, pre-scapula, axillary, inguinal, and popliteal lymph nodes. Examination of the lymph nodes is especially important in geriatric ferrets that may develop lymphoma. Obese animals may appear to have a lymphadenopathy when, in reality, the nodes palpate larger than normal because of excessive fat accumulation.

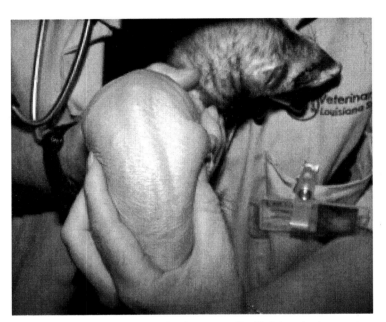

Figure 3-5 Alopecia. Ferrets can develop a generalized hair loss due to a number of disease processes. The most common disease presentation in which generalized hair loss occurs is adrenal disease.

Abdominal palpation is much more rewarding in ferrets compared with other mammals. The spleen, kidneys, and urinary bladder are readily palpated in the ferret. Splenomegaly is a common finding in ferrets and should be pursued with further diagnostics.

A neurological examination should also be performed, especially in animals with a history of weakness, paresis, or paralysis. The limbs of the animal should be thoroughly palpated to rule out fractures. The range of motion of the shoulder, elbow, carpus, pelvis, stifle, hock, and digits should be evaluated and any crepitace or problems recorded.

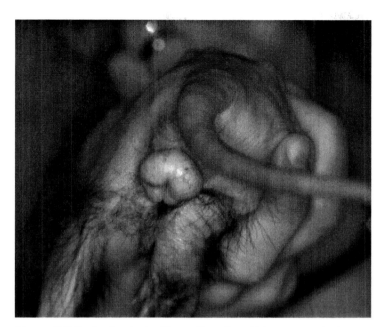

Figure 3-6 Swollen ferret vulva. The swollen vulva, which may occur due to hormonal influence, can become very prominent.

The anus should be evaluated and the perianal region should be free of fecal staining. The vulva of the neutered jill should be small (< 2 mm) and free of discharge or staining. Jills that are intact or have adrenal disease may develop an enlarged and turgid vulva (Figure 3-6). Often these animals will have a purulent vulvar discharge. The penis of the hob may be difficult to extract from the prepuce in an animal that is awake. If there is a history of stranguria, hematuria, or anuria, the animal should be sedated to thoroughly examine the penis.

Auscultation of the heart and lungs is an important component of the physical examination. In most mammals, the heart is located at approximately the point of the elbow, whereas in the ferret the heart is located in the mid-thoracic region between ribs 6–8. Placement of the stethoscope bell housing in the appropriate location is vital to evaluating the heart. The ferret heartbeat is much more rapid than domestic mammals and a sinus arrhythmia is a common finding.

Checking the rectal temperature of a ferret can be a real challenge. A digital thermometer is preferred over a glass thermometer because of the risk of breakage and injury to the animal. The ferret's normal body temperature should be between 100–103°F. Animals that struggle during the examination may have a falsely elevated body temperature.

After the examination is completed, the abnormal findings should be recorded and a problem list with differential diagnoses should be established. Based on the top differential diagnoses, diagnostic tests are prioritized to confirm diagnosis or to determine the severity of the disease.

DIAGNOSTIC SAMPLING

BLOOD COLLECTION

Obtaining a blood sample from a ferret may prove challenging at first; but with experience, the procedure will become routine. Ferrets that are not effectively immobilized using simple restraint should be anesthetized. The advent of inhalant anesthetics in veterinary medicine has simplified this procedure, allowing for rapid induction and recovery. The site of venipuncture will primarily depend upon the volume of sample required and the technician's skill level. Most clinical laboratories can perform complete blood counts and serum chemistry analysis on 1–2 ml of blood, significantly reducing the volume of blood required for testing. In certain cases, such as a blood transfusion, a larger volume of blood may need to be collected. The blood volume of the ferret has been estimated to be between 5–6% of the animal's body weight, and up to 10% of the animal's blood volume (5–6 ml/kg of body weight) may be safely collected at one time.[4]

A number of different venipuncture sites have been described to collect blood samples from the ferret. The volume that may be collected and the quality of the sample may vary from site to site. In general, the anterior venae cavae and jugular veins are the preferred sites for sample collection because large volumes of blood can be collected relatively easily. Other sites include the cephalic and saphenous veins and the tail artery. The cephalic veins should be reserved for intravenous catheterization and only used for venipuncture as a last resort. Clipping a nail to collect a blood sample has been recommended, but should not be performed because it is painful and yields lymph-diluted samples.

To collect a sample from the anterior venae cavae, place the animal in dorsal recumbency. A total of three people will be required to collect the sample if the animal is not anesthetized: two handlers and one sample collector. One handler

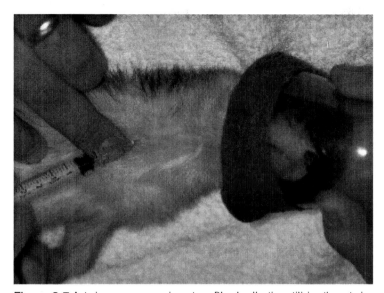

Figure 3-7 Anterior vena cava venipuncture. Blood collection utilizing the anterior vena cava provides ready access to large volumes of blood.

should grasp the head and stretch it forward with one hand, while using his/her second hand to pull the front legs back. The second handler should restrain the rear legs. Animals that struggle during the restraint should be anesthetized before performing the procedure. The landmarks for the venipuncture site are the manubrium and first left rib. The site should be aseptically prepared using an appropriate disinfectant to prevent the introduction of bacterial contaminants into the thorax. A 25-gauge needle fastened to a 3-ml syringe should be used to collect the sample (Figure 3-7). The needle should be inserted at a 45° angle to the body at the juncture of the manubrium and first left rib and directed toward the opposite rear leg. The level of the anterior vena cava may vary from animal to animal. Apply negative pressure to the syringe once the needle has entered the thorax until blood fills the syringe. In cases where a large volume of blood is required, such as for a transfusion, a 25-gauge butterfly catheter may be attached to a 12- or 20-ml syringe to facilitate collection.

The jugular vein should also be considered when large volumes of blood are required. There are two restraint techniques that may be used to prepare an animal for jugular venipuncture. The first technique is similar to that described for cats, where the animal's front legs are held over the edge of the table and the neck is stretched up. The second technique is performed on an animal in dorsal recumbency and restrained using the same technique described for the anterior venae cavae technique. Animals that are difficult to manually restrain should be anesthetized. The jugular vein of the ferret courses in a more lateral direction than in dogs and cats. Shaving the hair over the ventral cervical area may facilitate visualization of the vein; however, the ferret jugular vein is often surrounded by fat and difficult to visualize. The site should be aseptically prepared using an appropriate disinfectant. A 22-, 23-, or 25-gauge needle fastened to a 3-ml syringe may be used to collect the blood sample. The trachea is located on the ventral midline of the cervical region and may be used as a landmark. Apply gentle pressure with your thumb at the thoracic inlet to increase resistance in the vein and visibility. A slight bend (20° angle) in the needle may be made to improve access to the vein. The skin in the cervical region is more difficult to penetrate than in other regions of the body, therefore, be prepared to exert additional force. In those cases where the jugular vein is not visible, a "blind stick" will be necessary. The needle should be gently inserted into the vicinity of the jugular vein until a flash of blood is identified in the hub of the needle. Do not be overly aggressive when "searching" for the jugular, as there are other vital tissues in the cervical area that could become damaged.

The cephalic and saphenous veins may be used to collect small volumes of blood (<0.5 ml), but should be reserved for intravenous catheter sites. The cephalic vein is located over the ante-brachium, as in dogs, although the vein courses more laterally in the ferret (Figure 3-8). The lateral saphenous vein can be located above the hock and courses diagonally in an anterior to posterior fashion (Figure 3-9). Shaving the hair over the venipuncture sites will facilitate visibility. The site should be aseptically prepared using an appropriate disinfectant. The ferret should be restrained using the same techniques used to restrain a cat when collecting a blood sample from the cephalic or saphenous vein. A 25- or 26-gauge needle fastened to a 3-ml syringe may be used to collect the sample.

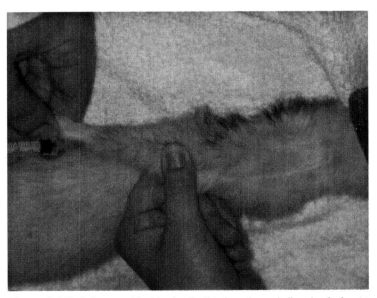

Figure 3-8 Technique used for blood collection from the cephalic vein of a ferret.

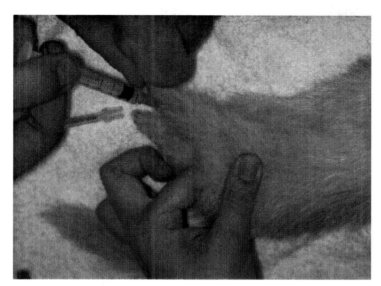

Again, a slight bend (20° angle) in the needle may simplify the approach to the vessel.

Blood samples may also be collected from the tail artery, although this technique is rarely used. The tail artery is located 2–3 mm deep to the midline of the ventral tail. The animal should be restrained by scruffing and pulling the legs caudally. The site should

Figure 3-9 Technique used for blood collection from the lateral saphenous vein of a ferret.

be aseptically prepared using an appropriate disinfectant. A 22-gauge needle fastened to a 3- or 6-ml syringe may be used. The needle should be inserted into the ventral midline of the tail and negative pressure applied until blood is observed filling the syringe. Because this is an artery, direct digital pressure should be applied to the site for a minimum of 3 minutes after withdrawing the needle.

Observed reference ranges for the ferret complete blood count (CBC) and serum chemistry panel are listed in Tables 3-2 and 3-3. These values represent observed reference ranges and should not be considered complete.

BONE MARROW ASPIRATION

There are several diseases that ferrets may develop that can lead to a suppression of the progenitor cells of the bone marrow, including estrogen induced anemia, neoplasia, and adrenal gland disease. Animals with a non-regenerative anemia, thrombocytopenia, leukopenia, or pancytopenia are good candidates for this diagnostic procedure.

There are a number of sites that can be used to collect a bone marrow sample (humeral, femur, iliac crest); however, the proximal femur is the most frequently used site because of accessibility. The ferret should be provided general anesthesia for the procedure. The animal should be placed into lateral recumbency and the area over the proximal femur shaved. The site should be aseptically prepared using an appropriate disinfectant and the procedure should be performed using sterile techniques. An incision (#15 scalpel blade) should be made over the greater trochanter of the femur. A 20- or 22-gauge 1–1.5" spinal needle may be inserted into the femur to collect the sample. A 6-ml syringe may be fastened to the spinal needle to aspirate the sample.

SPLENIC ASPIRATE

Splenomegaly is a common finding in adult ferrets. A splenic aspirate is a relatively noninvasive technique that may be used to collect a sample for cytology. Animals that are fractious should be anesthetized to prevent splenic laceration. The ferret should be restrained in right lateral recumbency and the left side of the body wall in the area of the spleen should be shaved and aseptically prepared. This procedure will introduce a needle into the abdomen, so it is vital that sterile techniques are followed closely. The spleen can be immobilized by grasping it through the skin and holding it between the thumb and index finger. A 25-gauge needle fastened to a 3-ml syringe may be used to collect the sample. The needle should be inserted into the spleen and negative pressure applied by rapidly pulling the plunger back several times. The needle should be removed from the spleen and the sample prepared for cytology. Remember that the sample is in the needle and pulling back on the plunger, once the needle is removed from the spleen, can result in the sample being pulled into the syringe and lost. Always remove the needle from the syringe, then pull air into the syringe, refasten the needle, and spray the sample onto microscope slides.

URINE COLLECTION AND INTERPRETATION

The collection of uncontaminated urine is essential to evaluating the true status of a sample. Free-catch urine samples are often contaminated with bacteria and may be misinterpreted by the novice. Fortunately, cystocentesis can be performed relatively easily on an unanesthetized ferret. The animal should be placed in dorsal recumbency and ventral abdomen aseptically prepared. The urinary bladder is located cranial to the pelvis and should be identified prior to attempting this procedure. Using your index finger and thumb, gently grasp the abdomen in the area of the bladder and move your hand in a cranial to caudal motion. The urinary bladder should palpate like a water filled balloon. A 25-gauge needle fastened to a 3- or 6-ml syringe may be used to collect the sample. Isolate the bladder between your index finger and thumb and insert the needle perpendicular to the body wall. Maintain a steady hand and prevent excessive movement of the needle within the abdomen.

Urinary catheterization may also be used to collect a urine sample, but is difficult in ferrets. Anesthesia will be required to perform this procedure. In the female, the urethral opening is located approximately 1 cm cranial to the clitoral fossa.[8] A vaginal speculum may be used to visualize the urethral opening and introduce an appropriate catheter (e.g., 3.5 French). In the male, the penis must be gently exteriorized from the prepuce. An appropriate catheter may be introduced into the urethra and sutured to the skin to maintain urethral patency.

Ferret urine should be yellow in color and have little turbidity (Table 3-4). These animals are true carnivores and should have a urine pH between 6.5–7.5.[9] Animals with alkaline urine may be predisposed to calculi formation. There should be no blood or bacteria from a sample collected via cystocentesis or catheterization.

Table 3–4
Urinalysis Results in the Ferret[6]

	Male	**Female**
Color	yellow	yellow
Turbidity	minimal	minimal
Volume (ml/24h)	26 (8–48)	28 (8–140)
Sodium (mmol/24h)	1.9 (0.4–6.7)	1.5 (0.2–5.6)
Potassium (mmol/24h)	2.9 (1.0–9.6)	2.1 (0.9–5.4)
pH	6.5–7.5	6.5–7.5
Protein (mg/dl)	7–33	0–32

MICROBIOLOGY

Ferrets are susceptible to potentially opportunistic Gram-positive or Gram-negative pathogen. Kits and geriatric animals are typically more susceptible to bacterial pathogens than a healthy adult animal. Animals being maintained on immunosuppressive doses of corticosteroids are also more susceptible to opportunistic infections. Sample collection should follow standard sterile techniques. A commercial sterile culturette and transport media (Culturette, Beckton Dickinson, Sparks, MD) may be used to collect samples and protect them from desiccation during transport to a diagnostic laboratory. Standard microbial techniques may be employed to isolate a potential pathogen. Most opportunistic infections are associated with aerobic infections; however, in certain abscesses facultative or obligate anaerobic organisms should be considered. *Helicobacter mustelae* are Gram-negative rods that are routinely cultured from gastric ulcers. Most bacterial infections are associated with pneumonia, urinary cystitis, and diarrhea. A number of pathogens have been isolated from these different organ systems, including *Streptococcus zooepidemicus* and *S. pneumoniae*, *E. coli*, *Klebsiella*, *Pseudomonas*, and *Bordetella*. Fungal infections in ferrets are rare. In cases where a fungal infection suspected, the techniques used to collect and process samples employed in other domestic species may be followed.

RADIOLOGY

Radiographs serve as an important diagnostic tool in ferret medicine. Standard safety protocols should be employed when radiographing ferrets. Ferrets should be anesthetized to ensure that quality radiographs are taken. Isoflurane is the anesthetic of choice. A ferret radiographic technique chart should be established based upon a facility's radiographic machine. A high capacity radiographic unit capable of producing 300-milliampere exposures at times of at least 1/60th of a second is recommended. The kVp settings should be adjustable by increments of 2 to provide finite detail. A thorough understanding of ferret anatomy is essential to radiographic interpretation.

PARASITOLOGY

Ear mites (*Otodectes cynotis*) are a common finding in ferrets, especially kits. Animals with ear mites will often present with a thick, brown discharge in the ear. Owners often complain that the animal shakes and scratches at its ears. A cotton-tip applicator dipped in mineral oil may be used to collect a sample from the ear for diagnosis. The sample should be placed onto a glass slide and evaluated under light microscopy.

Fleas that parasitize dogs and cats may also prey on ferrets. Ferrets with a flea infestation will often present with a history of pruritis and tail base alopecia. On close examination of the animal, the fleas or their feces ("flea-dirt") will be obvious. Kits or severely compromised adult animals may become severely anemic if they have a heavy flea burden. In these cases, a minute blood sample (<0.1 ml) may be collected and a packed cell volume determined. Animals with a packed cell volume less than 15% may require a blood transfusion. Flea eradication is similar to cats, and the owner should be aware of the importance of treating both the animal and the environment.

Ferrets maintained outdoors may be susceptible to fly strike, especially if they have a skin laceration. Animals maintained outdoors should be monitored closely for any injuries and the animal provided shelter and protection against flies. Animals that develop a maggot infestation should have the site shaved, maggots removed, and a topical antiseptic cream applied to protect the injury site.

Gastrointestinal parasitism is uncommon in ferrets. Ferrets allowed to play outdoors are more likely to develop a patent parasite infection than animals maintained indoors. A fecal sample should be submitted for a saline direct smear and a fecal float for kits at the time of their initial examination and for adult animals on an annual basis.

Ferrets are susceptible to *Dirofilaria immits,* and animals in heartworm endemic areas should be tested and given a heartworm preventative. Diagnosis of heartworm disease in ferrets can be difficult. The two most commonly used diagnostic tests in veterinary clinical practice are the Knott's test and the enzyme-linked immunosorbent assays (ELISA). The Knott's test is used to diagnose circulating microfilaria, and the ELISA test is used to diagnose circulating antigens produced by gravid female worms. Sensitivity of these tests is often lower in ferrets than in canids, because adult worm burdens are low (e.g., 1 worm) or occult (e.g., same sex). With the limitations of the currently available heartworm tests, echocardiography may provide a more definitive and consistent approach to heartworm disease diagnosis in the ferret.

Treatment of heartworm disease in the ferret is equally difficult. Most of the problems encountered with treatment are related to thromboembolism. The current treatment recommendation is Caparsolate (2.2 mg/kg IV q12h for 2 days) combined with an antithrombocytic drug.[10] Approximately one month after successful adulticide treatment, the animal should be placed on preventative therapy.[10]

VACCINATIONS

Canine distemper virus (CDV) is associated with high mortalities in affected ferrets. Ferret owners should be made aware of the risks of this disease and the likelihood of exposure, even to indoor animals. Vaccination is the best protection against infection. There is one USDA-approved vaccine (Fervac-D, United Vaccine, Madison, WI). The vaccine should be administered subcutaneously in the area between the shoulder blades. **Never use a canine combination or ferret cell origin vaccine, as these vaccines may induce the disease.** Vaccine reactions to this and other vaccines have been reported, but these reports are unsubstantiated. Ferrets that experience a hypersensitivity reaction may develop gastrointestinal signs, including vomiting and diarrhea, becoming dyspneic, and/or developing other systemic signs (e.g., depression, lethargy, and erythematous skin). Treatment of a ferret experiencing a vaccine reaction should follow the standard protocol for mammals and include diphenhydramine hydrochloride (Benadryl, Parke-Davis, Morris Plains, NJ) at 0.5–2.0 mg/kg, IM or IV.[4] Animals that have had a previous vaccine reaction should be pre-medicated with diphenhydramine hydrochloride 15 minutes prior to the vaccination. The standard CDV vaccine protocol for a kit should include a vaccine at 6 weeks, 10 weeks, and 14 weeks. A booster vaccine should be administered annually to adult animals.

Ferrets are susceptible to rabies and should be vaccinated against this devastating disease. There is one USDA-approved vaccine (Imrab 3, Rhone-Merieux Inc., Athens, GA.). The rabies vaccine should be administered to a kit at 12–14 weeks of age and a booster administered annually. The vaccine may be administered subcutaneously or intramuscularly and should follow local rabies ordinances. Vaccinated ferrets are currently protected under the same statutes as dogs and cats, whereas an unvaccinated animal should be managed as a wild animal. **Ferret owners should be made aware that, by law, unvaccinated animals that bite a human are supposed to be euthanized and tested for rabies.**

THERAPEUTICS

There are no approved therapeutics for the ferret in the United States. Current recommendations should follow those described for cats. The same routes of administration apply, including per os (PO), subcutaneous (SC), intramuscular (IM), intraosseus (IO), and intravenous (IV). Animals that are critical require routes of administration that provide rapid drug delivery, such as IM, IO or IV, whereas less critical animals may be given therapeutics PO or SC. Intravenous injections should be administered through an intravenous catheter. The preferred site for intravenous catheterization is the cephalic vein. Intramuscular injections are routinely administered into the epaxial muscles along the spine or in the limbs. The muscle masses of the ferret limb are relatively small in comparison to other mammals; therefore, the volume of the injection should be limited. Ferrets are very difficult to pill. There are a number of commercial compounding pharmacies that can compound a therapeutic into a liquid and simplify administration.

Fluid administration protocols for ferrets should follow those described for dogs and cats. Animals that are mildly dehydrated (<5%) may be administered fluids per os or subcutaneously, whereas an indwelling intravenous catheter should be placed in any animal that is greater than 5% dehydrated. Per os fluids should not be administered to any animal with gastrointestinal disease. Subcutaneous fluids may be administered in the subcutaneous space between the shoulder blades. The cephalic and lateral saphenous veins are routine sites for catheter placement. Ferrets that are alert and responsive will require sedation for this procedure, which may be accomplished by masking the animal with isoflurane anesthesia. A moribund animal will likely not require sedation. The animal should be placed in sternal recumbency for cephalic catheter placement, while the animal may be placed into lateral recumbency for lateral saphenous catheterization. One individual will need to "hold-off" the vessel by grasping the animal at the elbow for the cephalic vein and above the hock for the lateral saphenous. Intravenous catheters often become damaged when they are inserted through tough skin. To avoid this problem, make a puncture in the skin lateral to the vessel using a 22-gauge needle. A heparinized 24- to 26-gauge catheter may be introduced into the skin puncture and threaded into the vessel. An injection port should be fastened to the catheter and the device may be secured to the leg using tissue glue and appropriate bandage material. Ferrets that are very active and chew at the catheter may require an Elizabethan collar, which is commercially available or it may be fashioned from exposed radiographic film. The catheter should be flushed regularly (e.g., q4h) with 0.9% heparinized saline. The animal should be observed regularly to ensure the catheter remains patent and the animal does not become entangled in its fluid line.

Blood transfusions may be required in animals with severe anemias (PCV < 15%). Because ferrets lack distinct blood groups, they may be used as universal donors. Blood may be collected from an anesthetized blood donor from either the jugular vein or anterior vena cava using a 23-gauge butterfly catheter fastened to a 6- or 12-ml syringe. The syringe should be pre-loaded with an anticoagulant (e.g., acid-citrate-dextrose) at a ratio of 1-ml of anticoagulant to 6-ml of blood.[11] The blood should be administered to the recipient animal via a syringe pump or slow bolus through a cephalic or jugular catheter. The animal should be observed for any reactions to the transfusion. The volume of blood that may be collected from the donor and the volume required by the recipient may be determined using the formulae described in small animal medicine.

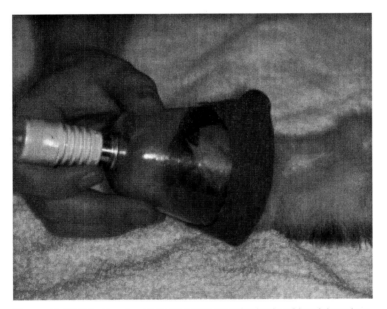

Figure 3-10 "Masking down." Ferret anesthetic induction is achieved through an induction chamber or a facemask (as shown).

SURGICAL AND ANESTHETIC ASSISTANCE

Ferrets may be anesthetized with a number of different agents (Table 3-5). Ferrets should fast for a minimum of 4 hours prior to an anesthetic procedure, although special precautions should be taken (e.g., IV dextrose) for an animal susceptible to a hypoglycemic episode (e.g., insulinoma ferret). Ferrets should be maintained on a water recirculating heating pad during any anesthetic procedure and recovered in a warmed environment to prevent hypothermia.

Table 3–5
Injectable Analgesic and Anesthetic Dosages for the Ferret[12]

Drug	Dose	Comments
Ketamine (Fox)	10–20 mg/kg IM 30–60 mg/kg IM	Tranquilization Anesthesia
Ketamine and Acepromazine (Hillyer)	20–25 mg/kg (K) IM 0.2–0.35 mg/kg (A) SC, IM	Anesthesia
Ketamine and Diazepam (Hillyer)	10–20 mg/kg (K) IM 1–2 mg/kg (D) IM	Anesthesia
Ketamine and Xylazine (Hillyer)	10–25 mg/kg (K) IM 1–2 mg/kg (X) IM	Anesthesia, avoid in sick animals
Butorphanol (Brown)	0.1–0.5 mg/kg IM q12h	Analgesia
Buprenorphine (Heard)	0.01–0.03 mg/kg SC, IM q12h	Analgesia

For short procedures, such as venipuncture or radiography, inhalant anesthesia may be used on a fractious animal. Ferrets may be "masked-down" using an appropriately sized mask or placed into a tank and anesthetized (Figure 3-10). Animals should be gradually anesthetized, starting at 1–2% and slowly increasing the concentration of the gas until a desired effect is achieved. Once the animal is anesthetized, it should be intubated using a 2.0 to 4.0 mm O.D. endotracheal tube. A laryngoscope may be used to increase visualization of the glottis. The animal should be monitored closely during the procedure using appropriate equipment (e.g., doppler, pulse oximeter, and ECG). Injectable anesthetics may be used to pre-anesthetize the animal or utilized in situations where an inhalant anesthetic is not available. There is some variation between the injectable anesthetics.

Surgical preparation of the ferret should follow the same protocols described for dogs and cats. The surgical site should be shaved using a standard grooming clipper at a slow, cautious speed to prevent clipper burn and tearing of the skin. The shaved area should be uniform and provide the surgeon ample room to perform the surgery without the risk of contamination. The surgical site should be aseptically prepared using a surgical scrub and warmed sterile saline. Avoid using alcohol to prepare the surgical site because it can result in significant heat loss. The surgical site should be covered with a sterile drape until the surgeon begins. The surgical instruments used to perform surgery on dogs and cats may be used for ferrets.

DISEASES

GASTROINTESTINAL DISEASES

Ingestion of Foreign Bodies

The curious nature of the ferret, in combination with its voracious appetite, is likely the reason why it ingests foreign material. Ferrets should always be monitored closely when they are outside of a cage. Kits are notorious for ingesting any potential foreign material, including metal, paper, and plastic, while adults are more likely to develop trichobezoars. Affected ferrets may exhibit lethargy, inappetence, vomiting, or diarrhea. Ferrets suspected of ingesting a foreign body should be thoroughly evaluated by performing a physical examination and survey radiographs. A contrast series may be necessary if the suspected foreign material is not evident on survey radiographs. Surgical correction is necessary to remove the foreign material. The surgical candidate should be stabilized prior to performing the procedure. The techniques used to remove a gastric foreign body (gastrotomy) or small intestine foreign body (enterotomy) should follow protocols described for domestic species.[13, 14]

Gastric ulcers are often reported in ferrets that experience chronic stress. There are a number of different etiologies that have been associated with gastric ulcers in the ferret, including primary gastritis, neoplasia, infection (e.g., *Helicobacter mustelae*), foreign body ingestion, and inappropriate drug use (e.g., corticosteroids). Ferrets that present with gastric ulcers are often inappetent, vomiting, and have melena or diarrhea. Many of these animals also grind their teeth and hypersalivate, symptoms which appear to be associated with upper gastrointestinal pain. Diagnosis of gastric ulcers should follow standard protocol. A complete blood count and serum chemistry panel should be performed to evaluate the animal's general health. Animals with chronic gastric ulcers may be anemic. Survey radiographs may be beneficial in identifying potential causes of the gastric ulcer. Endoscopy may be used to visualize the ulcers and collect biopsies for culture and histopathology. This technique is preferred when attempting to determine if an animal has *H. mustelae*. Ferrets should fast for at least 3 hours before performing radiographs or endoscopy to ensure no food remains in the stomach. Treatment for gastric ulcers depends on the specific diagnosis. In cases where a biopsy is not possible, empirical therapy is initiated that includes antibiotics (metronidazole and amoxicillin), an H_2 antagonist, and sucralfate (Carafate, Marion Merrell Dow, Inc., Kansas City, MO).

RESPIRATORY DISEASES

Ferrets are susceptible to many of the same opportunistic infections common to dogs and cats. Animals that develop clinical signs associated with respiratory disease, such as coughing, sneezing, and dyspnea, should undergo diagnostic testing in accordance with those described in other species.

Ferrets are susceptible to canine distemper virus (CDV) with mortalities approaching 100%. This virus replicates in the respiratory tract of the ferret and affected animals develop a chronic cough.[15] Ferrets with canine distemper may also develop symptoms associated with the skin (e.g., crusting under the chin and hyperkeratosis of the foot pads), eyes (e.g., blindness), and the central nervous system (e.g., incoordination). Treatment is unrewarding and affected animals should be humanely euthanized. Prevention may be achieved through routine vaccination.

Ferrets are susceptible to the human influenza virus. This virus primarily affects the upper respiratory system and clinically ill ferrets will often sneeze, cough, have difficulty smelling, and become inappetent and lethargic. Humans may infect their pets and vice versa. Affected animals should be provided supportive care and kept away from infants, the elderly, and those individuals with reduced immune function.

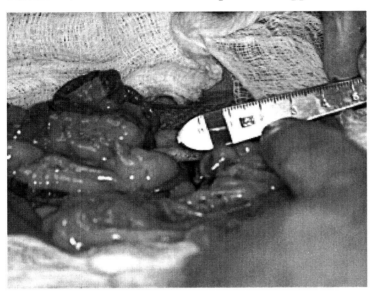
Figure 3-11 Insulinoma. Notice the neoplastic nodule within the pancreas.

NEOPLASIA

Neoplasia is a common finding in ferrets and may affect any age group.[16] The most common neoplastic diseases identified are adrenal gland adenoma, insulinoma, and lymphoma. There are a number of potential etiologies for the high incidence of neoplasia in ferrets, including genetics, early-age spay/neutering, diet, photoperiod, and infectious agents; but to date, no specific cause has been identified.

Adrenal gland disease is the most common neoplasia identified in adult ferrets. Affected animals often present with focal or generalized alopecia, pruritis, thinning of the skin, and weight loss. A majority of the animals remain active, and there appears to be no sex predilection—although hobs may develop prostatic disease, stranguria, and a return to sexual aggression, while a jill may develop a swollen vulva. In both genders a pancytopenia may develop. To diagnose adrenal gland disease, a series of diagnostic tests should be performed, including a complete blood count, chemistry panel, radiographs, ultrasound, and steroid hormone concentrations. Insulinomas are routinely identified in ferrets affected with adrenal gland disease (Figure 3-11). Current recommendations for treatment focus on surgical intervention, although some successful medical therapies have been reported. Performing an adrenalectomy does not guarantee remission of the neoplasia. Adrenal gland neoplasia is most commonly identified in the left adrenal gland, but may occur in both glands. Biopsy of the affected gland(s) should be performed. Adrenal gland hyperplasia, adenoma, or adenocarcinoma have been reported.

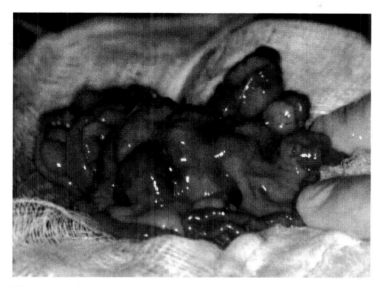

Figure 3-12 Lymphoma. Notice the enlarged mesenteric lymph node.

Insulinomas are another common tumor in adult ferrets. These beta-cell tumors may coalesce to form grossly visual nodules within the pancreas (Figure 3-12). Affected animals are often presented because they are glassy-eyed, have hind leg weakness, hypersalivate and paw at their mouths, and/or have seizures. Blood work, including a fasting blood glucose, insulin, complete blood count, and chemistry panel should be performed to confirm the diagnosis. If an animal is suspected of being hypoglycemic, then a fast is unnecessary. Survey radiographs and ultrasounds rarely prove to be diagnostic, but may be useful in identifying concurrent problems such as adrenal gland disease. Current recommendations for treatment are focused on surgical intervention, although medical therapies have been reported with some success. Performing a nodulectomy does not guarantee remission of the neoplasia. In cases where the neoplasia recurs, medical management using prednisone and diazoxide may be considered.

Lymphoma is the most common tumor in young ferrets.[15] Affected animals may be clinically normal or may present with weakness, lethargy, generalized lymphadenopathy, splenomegaly, and dyspnea. Diagnosis of lymphoma should include a complete blood count, chemistry panel, radiographs, ultrasound, and biopsy of affected tissues. Treatment can be difficult and remission is likely. There are a number of different chemotherapeutic protocols that may be used to treat an affected animal. The treatment protocol should be based upon the animal's condition and the owner's comfort level.

CARDIOVASCULAR DISEASE

Dilated and hypertrophic cardiomyopathies have been reported in ferrets. Affected animals are often presented with many of the same clinical signs reported in dogs and cats, including weakness, lethargy, dyspnea, exercise intolerance, and hind leg weakness. A full cardiac diagnostic series should be performed to assess the animal's condition and should include a complete blood count, serum chemistry profile, radiograph(s), echocardiograph and ECG. Medical management of the heart condition will vary depending upon the animal's general condition and the extent of the disease.

REPRODUCTIVE DISEASE

Ferrets are induced ovulators and an intact jill that is not bred may develop a life-threatening, estrogen induced anemia. An affected animal will have a history of being intact and not bred, developing a swollen vulva, pale mucous membranes, weakness and lethargy. A blood sample may be collected to assess the erythron and leukon. In most cases, a pancytopenia will develop. Prevention is key and any female ferret not being used for breeding should have an ovariohysterectomy performed.

UROGENITAL DISEASE

Ferrets may develop urolithiasis if they are maintained on a low quality cat food or dog food. Magnesium ammonium phosphate is the most common urolith identified in the ferret.[17] Cystitis may also be identified in animals with urolithiasis and should be managed accordingly. A thorough diagnostic screening should be performed on affected animals and should include a complete blood count, chemistry panel, radiograph(s), urinalysis, and urine culture. Affected animals often have an alkaline urine as a result of a predominance of plant based proteins in their diet, whereas an animal offered a high quality, meat-based diet will have an acidic urine (normal). Males that develop a blockage of the urethra should be considered an emergency and immediate steps taken to remove the offending calculi. In severe cases, surgical removal of the uroliths may be required.

Renal cysts are an incidental finding often reported at necropsy.[18] A specific etiology for renal cysts has not been determined. On occasion renal cysts will be identified on routine examination, survey radiographs, or ultrasound. A thorough diagnostic work-up, including an analysis of blood and urine, should be performed to determine if the animal has any renal compromise as a result of the renal cysts.

REFERENCES

1. Rupprecht, C.E., Gilbert, J., Pitts, R. et al., "Evaluation of an Inactivated Rabies Virus Vaccine in Domestic Ferrets," *Journal of the American Veterinary Medical Association* 193 (1990) 1614–1616.

2. Fox, J.G. "Taxonomy, History and Use." In Fox J.G. ed., *Biology and Diseases of the Ferret*. Philadelphia: Lea and Febiger, 1988: 3–13.

3. Brown, S.A. "Basic Anatomy, Physiology and Husbandry." In Hillyer, E.V. and Quesenberry, K.E. eds., *Ferrets, Rabbits and Rodents: Clinical Medicine and Surgery*. Philadelphia: W.B. Saunders, 1997: 3–13.

4. Fox, J.G. "Normal Clinical and Biological Parameters." In Fox, J.G. ed., *Biology and Diseases of the Ferret*. Philadelphia: Lea and Febiger, 1988: 159–73.

5. Bell, J. "Ferret Nutrition and Diseases Associated with Inadequate Nutrition," Proceeding of the North American Veterinary Conference, Orlando, FL, 1993: 719–720.

6. Thorton, P.C., Wright, P.A., Sacra P.J. et al., "The Ferret, *Mustela putorius furo*, as a New Species in Toxicology." *Lab Animals*, 13 (1979) 119–124.

7. Kawasaki, T.A. "Laboratory Parameters in Disease States in Ferrets," Proceedings of the North American Veterinary Conference, 1992: 663–7.

8. Quesenberry, K.E. "Basic Approach to Veterinary Care." In Hillyer, E.V. and Quesenberry, K.E. eds., *Ferrets, Rabbits and Rodents: Clinical Medicine and Surgery*. Philadelphia: W.B. Saunders, 1997: 14–25.

9. Williams, C.S.F. *Practice Guide to Laboratory Animals*. St. Louis: C.V. Mosby, 1976: 66.

10. Stamoulis, M.E. and Miller, M.S. "Cardiovascular Diseases." In Hillyer, E.V. and Quesenberry, K.E. eds., *Ferrets, Rabbits and Rodents: Clinical Medicine and Surgery*. Philadelphia: W.B. Saunders, 1997: 63–70.

11. Hoefer, H.L. "Transfusions in Exotic Species." In Hohenhaus A.E. ed., *Transfusion Medicine*. Philadelphia: J.B. Lippincott, 1992: 625–35.

12. Brown, S.A. "Ferret Drug Dosages." In Bauck, L., Boyer, T.H., Brown, S.A. et al., eds., *Exotic Animal Formulary*, Lakewood: American Animal Hospital Association, 1995: 5–11.

13. Orsher, R.J. and Rosin, E. "Small Intestine." In Slatter ed., *Textbook of Small Animal Surgery*. Philadelphia: W.B. Saunders, 1997: 593–612.

14. Van Sluys, F.J. "Gastric Foreign Bodies." In Slatter ed., *Textbook of Small Animal Surgery*. Philadelphia: W.B. Saunders, 1997: 568–71.

15. Pearson, R.C. and Gorham, J.R. "Viral Disease Models." In Fox, J.G. ed., *Biology and Diseases of the Ferret*. Philadelphia: Lea and Febiger, 1988: 305–14.

16. Brown, S.A. "Neoplasia." In Hillyer, E.V. and Quesenberry, K.E. eds., *Ferrets, Rabbits and Rodents: Clinical Medicine and Surgery*. Philadelphia: W.B. Saunders, 1997: 99–114.

17. Hillyer, E.V. "Urogenital Diseases." In Hillyer, E.V. and Quesenberry, K.E. eds., *Ferrets, Rabbits and Rodents: Clinical Medicine and Surgery*. Philadelphia: W.B. Saunders, 1997: 44–52.

18. Fox, J.G. "Systemic Diseases." In Fox, J.G. ed., *Biology and Diseases of the Ferret.* Philadelphia: Lea and Febiger, 1988: 255–73.

The following were not cited explicitly in the text

Fox, J.G. "Anesthesia and Surgery." In Fox, J.G., ed., *Biology and Diseases of the Ferret.* Philadelphia, Lea and Febiger, 1988: 289–30.

Heard, D.J. "Principles and Techniques of Anesthesia and Analgesia for Exotic Practice." *Vet Clinic of North Am/Small Animal Practice* 23, 1993: 1301–1327.

Hillyer, E.V. and Brown, S.A. "Ferrets." In Birchard, S.J. and Sherding, R.G. eds., *Saunders Manual of Small Animal Practice.* Philadelphia: W.B. Saunders, 1994: 1317–44.

CHAPTER 4

RABBITS

INTRODUCTION

One of the most common misconceptions regarding rabbits is that they belong to the order Rodentia, which includes mice, rats, and guinea pigs. Rabbits do not belong to the family Rodentia, but belong to the order of animals called Lagomorpha, which also includes hares and pikas. Rabbits differ from mice, rats, and guinea pigs because they have a second pair of underdeveloped incisor teeth directly behind the primary incisors, which rodents do not have. This classification difference is important to point out in the beginning of this chapter, because rabbit husbandry and health concerns are very different from those of rodents. Many rabbits are obtained through impulse purchases during the spring and Easter season. Often these impulse purchases do not include client education on proper husbandry, nutrition, or health maintenance. Hopefully, the new rabbit owner will schedule an appointment with a veterinarian for a routine health examination and, most importantly, receive an education during the visit on the requirements for maintaining a healthy, happy pet. Frequently, an owner will ask questions regarding basic physiologic values of their new pet rabbit. It is not only important for the technician to know the normal physiologic values to answer owners' questions, but also to assess the patients' health status upon presentation to the clinic and to administer medical therapy (Table 4-1).

Table 4–1
Rabbit Basic Information[1]

Body weight	Adult male (buck)	2–5 kg
	Adult female (doe)	2–6 kg
	Birth weight (bunny)	30–80 g
Temperature, pulse and respiration	Rectal body temperature	101.3–104°F
	Normal heart rate	180–250 beats/minute
	Normal respiratory rate	30–60 breaths/minute
Amounts of food and water	Daily food consumption	50 g/kg
	Daily water consumption	50–150 ml/kg
	Daily urine excretion	10–35 ml/kg
Age at onset of puberty and breeding life	Sexual maturity, male	22–52 weeks
	Sexual maturity, female	22–52 weeks
	Breeding life, males	60–72 months
	Breeding life, females	24–36 months
Female reproductive cycle	Estrous cycle	Induced ovulation
	Estrus duration	Prolonged
	Ovulation rate	6–10 eggs
	Pseudopregnancy	16–17 days
	Gestation length	30–33 days
	Litter size	4–12 bunnies

The technician needs to become familiar with a few areas of rabbit anatomy. It may seem that rabbits are very docile animals. Although rabbits can be very gentle, they are territorial and will mark and viciously defend their territory. The chin glands, anal glands, and inguinal glands are used to mark territory and young. Males mark most often, followed by dominates of both sexes over subordinates.1 The female may have a large "dewlap" or fold of skin under her chin. During nesting, the female sometimes removes hair from the dewlap as a source of soft nest material. Rabbits do not have footpads like cats, dogs, and rodents. Their feet are covered with fur that provides protection to the plantar surface of the foot. This fur has developed to protect the feet in the rabbit's natural habitat, not in wire-bottomed cages. Large, obese rabbits may develop sores on the ventral surface of the hock, since that part of the leg is in contact with the cage surface during rest. Owners and rabbit handlers must be cautious of the sharp claws, especially the claws on the rear legs. When struggling, a rabbit will kick forward with the rear legs and scratch, sometimes severely, an unprepared holder. It is not recommended to declaw rabbits. The underlying tissue support and footpads are not present to aid and protect the foot when healing. Sharp claws should be trimmed to blunt the sharp points, or the plastic rubberized Soft-Paws® may be used. The ears make up a large percentage of the body. At no time should the animal be picked up by the ears.

HUSBANDRY

ENVIRONMENTAL CONCERNS

Pet rabbits are very sensitive to heat. They have a well-developed hair coat that protects them against cold weather, but they quickly overheat when environmental temperatures are high. When a rabbit is housed outside, in a non-air-conditioned house, or apartment, or a car (when traveling), the owner must implement precautions. Common housing precautions against heat stress include: providing a shaded enclosure (roof or natural setting), placing the rabbit in an air-conditioned room during the summer months, and/or providing a fan for an animal housed outside. During the winter months, when humans need extra clothing, pet owners may erroneously assume that extra measures are needed to keep their pet rabbits warm. If a plywood "house" is placed in the animal's enclosure and lined with hay, this should protect the animal in temperatures down to 32°F (Figures 4-1A, 4-1B, and 4-1C).

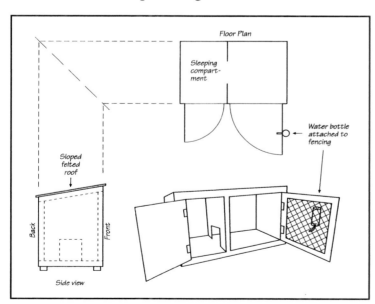

Figure 4-1A Typical outdoor housing for pet rabbits. The cage protects the rabbit from predators and inclement weather.

When educating a rabbit owner, emphasis must be placed on their pet's intolerance to heat. It would be most appropriate to give owners this information in the spring, when most of these pets are purchased.

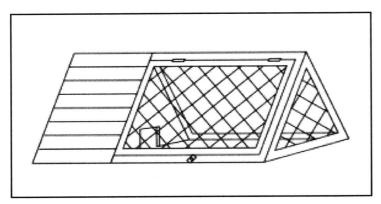

Figure 4-1B Morant pen. This outdoor hutch allows the rabbit access to the sun and grass, while providing shelter in the event of a storm.

Rabbit owners will house their pets either primarily inside or primarily outside. Animals that are housed inside can be allowed to roam outside in the grass within a fenced enclosure. No exposure to other animals such as dogs or cats is recommended because of the unpredictable nature of a natural hunter when a prey animal (the rabbit) is observed. If rabbits are allowed to roam the house, plants and electrical cords need to be removed or made inaccessible. These animals can maneuver behind furniture and "dig" under rugs, so hiding cords in this manner is unacceptable. The recommendation for allowing pet rabbits to roam free within a given area includes: (a) making it impossible for the rabbit to escape and (b) observing the animal while it is out of the cage. When outside, a special wire enclosure or grazing ark can be made with wire sides and top. The open bottom of the special enclosure allows the animal to graze protected and unattended. Because the grazing ark is mobile, the owner can move the enclosure to fresh grass as needed.

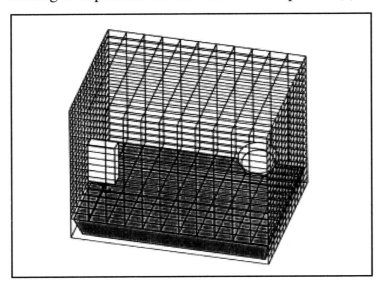

Figure 4-1C Indoor rabbit housing. This pop-up style rabbit hutch has a place for food and a water bottle.

Rabbits can be house-trained to use a litter tray. The tray should have low sides filled with cat litter, and, when first acquired, the new pet should be placed in the tray every few minutes.[1] Litter training is possible with most rabbits, but remember these animals are very territorial; and adult bucks may mark different areas of the house with strong smelling feces to identify their territory. These animals are prey species in their natural setting and propagate readily. Pet rabbits should not be housed together after they reach sexual maturity because of their strong territorial nature. It is not uncommon for two males housed together to viciously fight when they reach sexual maturity. Fighting can even occur when a male and female are housed together, with the female fighting the male rabbit in her territory. For breeding purposes, always bring the female rabbit into the male's enclosure for the act of breeding, and then return the doe to her cage.

Commercial cages are available to house rabbits indoors. These relatively small cages are excellent for the dwarf and mini breeds, but lack the exercise space needed for the larger breeds. If a rabbit cage is to be built, two functional spaces are needed: one space for resting and sleeping, and the other for exercise. As mentioned earlier, rabbits are susceptible to foot/leg problems (sore hocks) if they are large and are housed on a wire-bottom cage. The cage bottom must have a solid surface in part of the area, and the other section (which is usually wire) should be covered with a layer of substrate—either hay or large pine shavings. It is recommended that the owners clean the cage every one to two days. The sides of the cage must be made of wire to allow for ventilation. The top can be made of wire; but if the cage is outdoors, the area in which the rabbit sleeps needs to be covered with plywood or corrugated fiberglass-roofing material to protect against precipitation.

Since these animals are natural prey species, living with dogs and cats is a potential danger. At no time should the rabbit be allowed to commingle with dogs or cats, and if allowed out of their cage, only do so under supervision. There is no problem with housing rabbits with birds, but rabbits may carry a disease that is deadly to guinea pigs, *Bordetella bronchiseptica*.[1] Rabbits can carry this bacteria with no ill effects and transmit it to guinea pigs.

NUTRITION

Rabbits normally feed in the early morning and in the evening. They also eat their feces to reinoculate their digestive system with good bacteria. The process of eating feces is called coprophagy, and this usually occurs 3–8 hours after eating.[2] These soft and sweet smelling feces, or cecotropes, are often produced in the early hours of the morning. The cecotropes contain high levels of vitamin B and K and have twice the protein and half the fiber of regular hard feces.[3]

The most common feed offered to rabbits is alfalfa meal-based pellets. These pellets can be purchased with protein contents that range from 10–12% to 22–24%. Pellets containing 16% protein are the most commonly fed. Fiber content is recommended to be over 16% to guard against anorexia and diarrhea. A higher fiber content helps reduce the onset of obesity, which is a common presentation affecting pet rabbits. Free-choice feeding of pellets also encourages obesity; therefore, sedentary pet rabbits should be fed 1/8–1/2 cup per day, depending on their size.[3] The exception to this rule is with lactating does and growing young, which need as much food as they will eat. Wait five days after birth and have the owner start increasing the amount of pellets by 150 grams or 5 ounces per day.[3] If there are no pellets left in the food container over the next five-day period, add 150 grams more food. Reduce the amount of pellets in the diet only when excess remains the next morning. At weaning, it is recommended that the doe be removed from the cage to reduce the stress of a new environment on the young. Recently, there has been an emphasis on the importance of fiber in a rabbit's diet to prevent obesity, diarrhea, and hairballs. Timothy hay has been recommended as the best source for rabbit fiber. Unfortunately, timothy hay may not be available in many areas. Although there are claims that alfalfa hay may be too high in calcium, many rabbits have lived long, healthy lives on this fiber source. Overall, the best daily diet for pet rabbits is a measured alfalfa meal-based pellet with a hay supplement and a treat of dark green leafy vegetables or a free-choice hay diet, preferably timothy hay, with a vegetable supplement.[3]

Water is extremely important and access to clean tap water needs to be provided. Rabbits easily learn to drink from inverted water bottles that have a stainless steel tube extending down into the cage (Figure 4-2). These water containers are commonly sold as Lix-it® bottles. Rabbits, like most animals, drink from water bowls, but their low profile often contaminates the water bowl with food and feces. Drinking from the

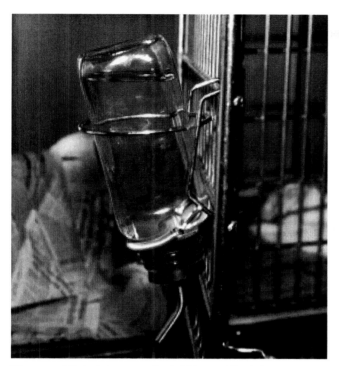

Figure 4-2 Typical sipper water bottle. This type of bottle is recommended for rabbit enclosures.

water bowl will also moisten the dewlap on large females, predisposing them to bacterial and fungal dermatitis. The water bottle must be kept clean and full of fresh water at all times.

HISTORY

A thorough history of the patient must be obtained before an educational recommendation can be given, or a proper physical exam performed. The name, breed, sex, and age of the animal to be examined are the first questions when taking a patient's history. As noted in Table 4-1, there is quite a difference in the physiologic parameters when comparing sex and rabbit breed. As with most species, smaller breeds of rabbits will mature faster than larger breeds. Common breeds of large pet rabbits are Angora, Lop-Eared, and New Zealand White; common small breeds are Mini Lop-Eared and Netherlands Dwarf (Figures 4-3A and 4-3B). The next group of questions centers on general background information such as length of time owned, where the animal was acquired, how often the animal is handled, and character of the fecal material. After these preliminary questions, you should start to have a basic understanding of the owner's knowledge of rabbits and care provided. Husbandry questions should follow, including: indoor/outdoor roaming habits, cage location, type and size of caging, cage substrate, frequency of cage cleaning, and the type of disinfectant (if any) that is used when cleaning the cage. Some of the most important questions you should ask a rabbit owner are: the type of food and water that is offered, and how much and how often the bowls are cleaned and refilled. The rabbit gastrointestinal system is very sensitive and rabbits are susceptible to obesity; therefore, educating clients in husbandry will help a pet rabbit reach its life expectancy. One area of questioning that must not be over-

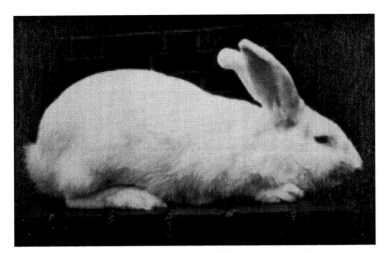

Figure 4-3A A New Zealand White. These rabbits have been popular pets and have been used in laboratory studies for many years.

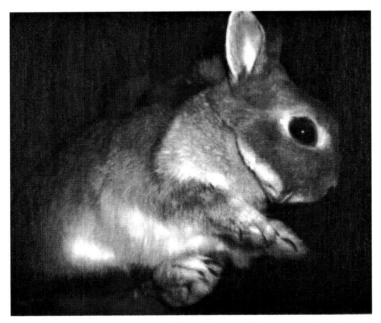

Figure 4-3B A Netherlands Dwarf. This rabbit, which is being properly held, can be identified by its small body conformation and ears.

looked is the status of other pets or animals in the house. Housing other pets with rabbits exposes all to disease and injury. Finally, the technician should obtain information about past health problems and the reason the patient is presenting.

Many larger breed rabbits may weigh up to 6 kilograms. The smaller breeds seem to be the most popular companion animals. Many unwanted older rabbits are large breed animals that were sold as bunnies, either unknowingly or unscrupulously, as a true dwarf breed. The owner who brings in a rabbit that he believes is a dwarf breed, but is not, should be informed of this potential surprise.

RESTRAINT

It is very difficult to restrain most rabbit patients. These small mammals have very strong muscles in their rear legs and jump quickly, with force. If not maintained in a proper position, a patient can jump out of the technician's arms onto the floor. An unexpected fall of this magnitude often creates an injury that was not present at the beginning of the appointment. To prevent this tragic scenario, there are certain guidelines to follow when holding a rabbit for examination, transportation, and placement in or removal from a cage.

Ears are not handles. Although rabbit ears are usually large and appear to be an excellent piece of anatomy to grasp, do not succumb to this illusion. The ears are delicate and when pulled a rabbit will use its powerful rear legs to escape. When a rabbit kicks its rear legs and its body is unsupported, spinal trauma may occur, which can cause temporary or permanent paralysis. Always support the body by placing a hand on the rear of the animal, during transport or examination (Figure 4-4). When removing the patient from a cage or pet carrier, grab the scruff with one hand, placing the other hand under its tail, supporting the rear legs. Place the animal on an examination table that is covered with a towel, which provides a

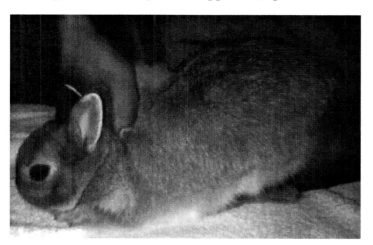

Figure 4-4 Proper holding. A rabbit should be properly held on the exam table by grabbing the scruff of the neck and supporting the rear legs.

nonslip surface. This towel can then be wrapped around the animal's body, forming a "bunny burrito," thus preventing leg movement (Figures 4-5A and 4-5B). While in a bunny burrito, the animal's head and tail areas can be examined and oral medications can be administered. The towel must be removed to perform a full body examination and auscultation. If the animal is transported, the head is placed in the crook of an elbow, with the arm supporting the body of the rabbit and the hand of that arm over

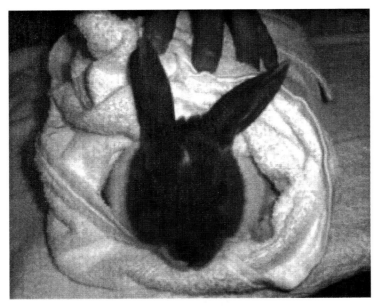

Figure 4-5A Frontal view. A bunny burrito is another form of rabbit restraint that utilizes a towel to prevent excess leg movement.

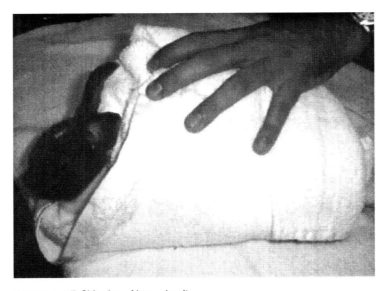

Figure 4-5B Side view of bunny burrito.

the rump. The opposite hand should grab the scruff of the neck (Figure 4-6). When placing a patient into a cage or carrier always back the animal into the enclosure. If rabbits are placed headfirst into an enclosure, they may jump out of a handler's grasp into the cage, possibly injuring themselves or the handler.

PHYSICAL EXAMINATION

The rabbit physical examination should always take place on a properly restrained animal. This is easier said than done on many rabbit patients, but veterinary technicians should heed this advice to prevent tragedies from occurring. Observation of the animal in the carrier initiates a physical examination. The animal's attitude, posture, and physical activity (if any) is observed and noted in the record. A close examination of the hair coat and skin is next, with the examiner looking for hair loss, skin lesions, and ectoparasites. Rabbits

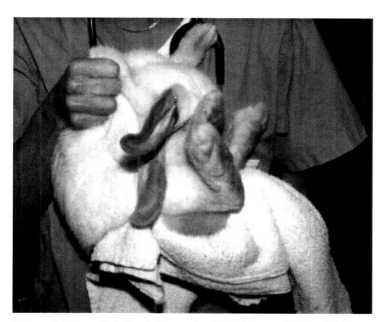

Figure 4-6 Proper technique to transport a rabbit. Make sure that the rabbit's rear legs are supported as the opposite hand has a firm grip on the scruff of the neck.

are susceptible to respiratory disease, ear mites, and ocular trauma. These disease problems must be considered during an external physical examination of the eyes, nose, and ears. One major problem rabbits often present with is malocclusion of the incisors and/or molars. Rabbit patients generally do not like people looking in their mouths, especially if they have dental problems. Proper restraint is emphasized for the oral examination. The lips can be manipulated with a tongue depressor allowing the examiner to observe the front teeth. Patients have been known to bite an unsuspecting veterinarian or technician during this procedure, so caution is called for. An easy way to examine the molars in the back of a rabbit's small mouth is to use an otoscope with an appropriate-sized head. This is about the only way to simplify a difficult operation. Hydration status of the animal may be checked during the oral examination through mucous membrane capillary refill time or packed cell volume percent, corneal moisture, or skin elasticity (skin tenting). Palpation of the body and extremities is necessary to look for possible fractures, and lymph node or organ enlargements. The examination should be completed with a neurologic assessment, auscultation of the heart and respiratory system, and examination of the external reproductive structures and anus.

After the examination is completed, any abnormal findings are recorded and a list of differential diagnoses is established. Based on the top differential diagnoses, diagnostic tests are prioritized to confirm a diagnosis or to determine the severity of the disease.

DIAGNOSTIC SAMPLING

BLOOD COLLECTION

Rabbits are difficult patients from which to obtain blood for diagnostic testing. In many older texts, the larger rabbit species were used as examples of how to collect blood from the marginal ear vein or central ear artery (Figure 4-7). In larger rabbit species, these sites are effective in obtaining blood at volumes necessary for the requested diagnostic tests; but this is not the case in the smaller, popular companion rabbit species. While the marginal ear vein and central ear artery may be considered in small rabbit breeds, they are often too small to collect any significant amount of blood. Other recommended venipuncture sites include the jugular vein (site of choice for smaller rabbit breeds), the cephalic vein, and the lateral saphenous vein. If the ear vein or artery is used for blood collection, the fur over the vessel must be plucked, and an alcohol wipe used to help with identification of the collection site. The vein or artery should be clamped with two fingers proximal to the venipuncture area to increase vascular pressure and dilate the vessel. A small gauge needle is used, 25-, 26-, or 27-gauge, to penetrate the ear artery or vein. If blood collection is slow due to vessel size, heperinized needles will help prevent blood clotting in the syringe. To circumvent collapse of the vein or artery from excess pressure during collection with a syringe or vacutainer tube, allow the blood to drip from a needle placed in the vessel, without a syringe attached into an open blood tube.[4] Rabbit skin is very elastic and thin, predisposing it to tears and abrasions when being clipped. Great care needs to

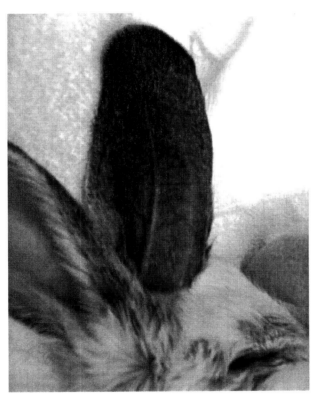

Figure 4-7 Marginal ear vein and central artery. These are commonly used for venipuncture and injection sites.

be followed when clipping rabbit fur, because of its thickness and the sensitive underlying skin. The ear vein and artery have a tendency to develop thrombi leading to vascular ischemia, which ultimately causes necrosis of the affected area on the dorsal surface of the ear. Possible ear trauma may occur any time that blood is collected from an ear vessel. Consideration of this potential injury should be used in determining the site of choice for venipuncture.

The cephalic veins are accessible, more so in larger breeds than smaller breeds, because of the short antebrachial length and small vein size in the diminutive rabbits. This is also true for the saphenous vein, which courses across the lateral aspect of the tibia. Another caution regarding shaving rabbit fur: remember to clean the clippers often to remove cut hair and gently clip hair close to the skin to prevent lacerations and abrasions.

The site of choice for blood collection in most rabbit species of varying sizes is the jugular vein. However, ear veins may also be used to collect blood, or they can be used for intravenous catheter placement. While some rabbit patients do not need sedation to obtain blood samples, it may be easier to provide a small amount of tranquilization to reduce stress and possible injury to the patient or personnel. Isoflurane, inhalation anesthesia (induction 5% then maintain at 1.5–2% with a 1.5 L flow rate of oxygen), administered through a facemask is probably the easiest, quickest, and safest method to sedate a rabbit for venipuncture and other diagnostic collection techniques. When collecting any diagnostic sample from a rabbit patient that is fractious, always consider sedation to prevent injury to the patient. The neck should be shaved from the mid-cervical to the caudal cervical area

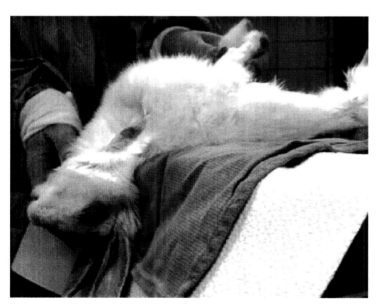

Figure 4-8 Proper venipuncture position for access to the rabbit jugular vein.

Table 4–2
Rabbit Complete Blood Count Reference Ranges

Erythrocytes	$4–4 \times 10^6/mm^3$
Hematocrit	36–48%
Hemoglobin	10.0–15.5 mg/dl
Leukocytes	$9–11 \times 10^3/mm^3$
Neutrophils	20–74%
Lymphocytes	30–85%
Eosinophils	0–4%
Monocytes	1–4%
Basophils	2–7%
Platelets	$250–270 \times 10^3/mm^3$
Serum protein	5.4–7.5 g/dl
Albumin	2.7–4.6 g/dl
Globulin	1.5–2.8 g/dl

Table 4–3
Rabbit Serum Biochemistry Reference Ranges

Serum glucose	75–150 mg/dl
Blood urea nitrogen	17.0–23.5 mg/dl
Creatinine	0.8–1.8 mg/dl
Total bilirubin	0.25–0.74 mg/dl
Serum lipids	280–350 mg/dl
Phospholipids	75–113 mg/dl
Triglycerides	124–156 mg/dl
Cholesterol	35–53 mg/dl
Serum calcium	5.6–12.5 mg/dl
Serum phosphate	4.0–6.2 mg/dl
Alkaline phosphatase	4–16 U/L
Alanine aminotransferase (ALT)	48–80 U/L
Aspartate aminotransferase (AST)	14–113 U/L
Lactic dehydrogenase	34–129 U/L

on the ventral, ventrolateral aspect of the body. To collect the blood, the rabbit should be placed in dorsal recumbency with the head over the edge of the table and the feet held in a caudal position (Figure 4-8). Take care not to overextend the neck in this position or respiratory compromise may occur. Even the smallest rabbit breeds have a large enough blood volume for safe collection to obtain diagnostic results. Rabbit blood volume has been published between 57–78 ml/kg.[5] Reference ranges for complete blood counts and serum chemistry panels are listed in Tables 4-2 and 4-3.[4,6,7]

BONE MARROW ASPIRATION

Recommended sites for collecting bone marrow in rabbits include the femur, humerus, pelvis, and proximal tibia. The technician should follow the same precollection protocol when obtaining a bone marrow aspirate in a rabbit as with any other small animal. The patient must be anesthetized for this procedure.

COLLECTION OF CEREBROSPINAL FLUID (CSF)

This is not a very common diagnostic procedure performed on pet rabbits, but it may be helpful in diagnosing listeriosis if the cerebrospinal fluid (CSF) is cultured.[5] CSF samples should be either submitted quickly or refrigerated to prevent cellular degradation, which occurs rapidly at room temperature. To position the patient correctly, the rabbit is placed in lateral recumbency with its head flexed to the ventral chest wall. The area from the occipital protuberance to the level of the third cervical vertebra and laterally past the margin of the atlas need to be prepped for the collection procedure.[4] This external skin preparation is similar to the methods used for CSF in canine patients. A 22-gauge, 1.5–3.5" spinal needle is recommended for this procedure in rabbits. A stylet is always recommended to prevent blockage of the needle in this very critical procedure. The spinal needle should enter the skin halfway between the cranial margins of the wings of the atlas and the occipital protuberance, slowly advancing toward the nose until penetration is felt through the dura and subarachnoid membranes.[5] The CSF should be allowed to drip into a plastic collection device, because leukocytes adhere to glass.[5] As with other companion animal species, the area being tested is surrounded by very vascular tissue and blood contamination of the CSF sample blood commonly occurs; therefore, the sample should be monitored for quality during collection.

URINE COLLECTION UTILIZING CYSTOCENTESIS

A cystocentesis can be successfully accomplished on most rabbit patients without sedation or anesthesia. Rabbits can be hypnotized while in dorsal recumbency, which is the position of choice for cystocentesis collection. The patient's scruff and rear limbs need to be restrained to prevent any sudden movements while the needle is in the bladder collecting urine. A 22-gauge needle attached to a 10-ml syringe is the recommended collection combination for cystocentesis. The bladder should be palpated cranial to the pelvis along the ventral midline of the body prior to placing the needle in the abdomen.[5] Cystocentesis preparation for rabbits is similar to dogs and cats. It is imperative that all precautions are considered to prevent an iatrogenic bladder infection.

Sedation with Midazolam, 0.5–2 mg/kg intramuscularly, will provide excellent sedation for catheterization of the urethra in male and female rabbits.[8] The male is collected with a well-lubricated 9 French catheter.[5] The patient is best positioned in a sitting posture to extend the penis and access the urethra. The female's urethral os is located on the floor of the vagina and is best catheterized in sternal recumbency.[5]

Normal rabbit urine ranges in color from orange to brown. The urine color corresponds to diet, concentration of crystals, and urinary tract health. Normal rabbit urine is cloudy, containing many ammonium magnesium phosphate, calcium carbonate monohydrate, and anhydrous calcium carbonate crystals. This finding is different from any other companion animal and should be recognized as a normal finding. In Table 4-4 the normal parameters of a rabbit urinalysis are listed.[8]

MICROBIOLOGY

Rabbits are predisposed to *Pasteurella multocida* infections that usually present as respiratory disease. *P. multocida* are so common in rabbits that it is often called "snuffles" because of the nasal and ocular discharge associated with the disease. To culture the organism for isolation, a mini-tipped culturette is introduced into the deep nasal sinuses to the level of the medial canthus of the eye.[5] If the rabbit is too fractious, sedation is recommended. Abscesses that may or may not be caused by *P. multocida, Staphylococcus aureus, Pseudomonas aeruginosa, Proteus* species, and *Bacteroides* species have to be cultured on the interior wall of the lesion because most rabbit abscesses are sterile in the center. All other culture procedures used to collect fungal and bacterial organisms in rabbit patients are similar to those employed on dogs and cats.

RADIOLOGY

There are many rabbit case presentations that require radiographic evaluation, including fractures, malocclusion, internal abscesses, and reproductive, gastrointestinal, and respiratory diseases. It is recommended to sedate or maintain the patient under general anesthesia for the radiographic procedure. This prevents injury and stress to the patient

Table 4-4
Rabbit Normal Urinalysis Values

Urine volume	
Large	20-350 ml/kg/day
Average	130 ml/kg/day
Specific gravity	1.003-1.036
Average pH	8.2
Crystals present	Ammonium magnesium phosphate, calcium carbonate monohydrate, calcium anhydrous carbonate
Casts, epithelial cells, or bacteria	Absent to rare
Leukocytes or erythrocytes present	Occasional
Albumin present	Occasional in young rabbits

and usually prevents poor radiographic images due to movement of the patient. Most importantly, it reduces the chance of human skeletons (hands and fingers) from showing up in the film. Isoflurane is the general anesthesia of choice for rapid induction and recovery.

PARASITOLOGY

Ectoparasites

Psoroptes cuniculi, or the rabbit ear mite, is a very common finding in pet rabbits (Figure 4-9A). The animal usually presents with thick crust originating from the base of the external ear canal extending up to, and sometimes out of, the ventral aspect of the pinna (Figure 4-9B). Identification of the mite can be made through a direct examination of the ear crust or observation of the mites within the ear canal using an otoscope. Treat with ivermectin (Ivomec, Merck AgVet Division, Rahway, NJ) at 400 µg/kg SC once every 2 weeks for three treatments, or once and repeated in 18 days.[9] The crusts should not be cleaned because the underlying tissue is very irritated. Once the mites have been killed and healing takes place, the crust usually sloughs in one piece. Topical treatment of the infestation is not necessary if ivermectin is being used,

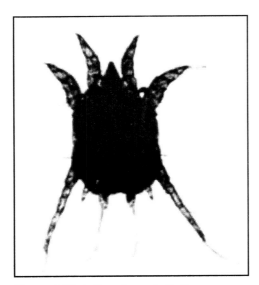

Figure 4-9A A *Psoroptes cuniculi* mite.

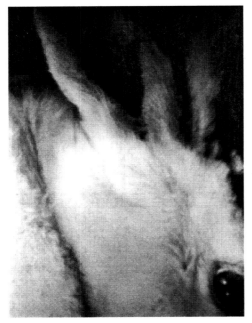

Figure 4-9B *Otitis externa.* This is caused by an infestation of rabbit ear mites *(Psoroptes cuniculi).*

but it may help as adjunct therapy to expedite the healing process.

Cheyletiella parasitovorax is commonly called walking dandruff, or the rabbit fur mite. This ectoparasite can also infect humans and other companion animals. *C. parasitovorax* is rather large, and the dandruff and debris that are collected off of a suspect case can be examined under a microscope by picking up the material on a piece of scotch tape. This is commonly called "The Scotch Tape" test in dermatology. The life cycle of the rabbit fur mite is about 5 weeks, and ivermectin is the treatment of choice. The pet's environment should also be treated with flea control products to prevent re-exposure. Other mites have been diagnosed in rabbits, including *Sarcoptes scabiei, Notoedres cati* and *Demodex cuniculi*; but these are relatively uncommon findings.[9]

Fleas also feed on rabbits. As with other companion animals, signs of infestation include: dried bloody flea feces ("flea dirt"), an itching patient, and the appearance of fleas themselves. Treatment is similar to cats, and the owner must be reminded to treat the environment also.[9]

Large maggot larvae and smaller fly larvae affect rabbits. The large maggot larvae from flies (*Cuterebra* spp.) are usually noted as a swelling in the ventral cervical, axillary, or inguinal area or the dorsal rear.[9] Maggots must be surgically removed and surrounding tissues treated to prevent any secondary complications. Smaller fly larvae are attracted to moist, matted fur around the anogenital area. The patient that is suffering from maggot infestation needs to have the fur trimmed and skin treated. The cleaning and removal of maggots is best accomplished on a sedated patient.

Internal parasites

The most common intestinal parasite class that affects rabbits is coccidia of the genus *Eimeria*. *E. stiedae*, which affects the liver, is very common in mismanaged rabbit breeding operations. All other rabbit coccidia affect the intestinal tract with diarrhea being the most common clinical presentation. Coccidia, protozoan parasites, nematode, cestode, and trematode parasites can be diagnosed through direct fecal examinations and fecal flotations. Once the parasite has been correctly identified, the appropriate medication should be prescribed.

THERAPEUTICS

Often rabbit patients do not present in a condition that would initially seem critical. After a thorough history and physical examination, the veterinarian may decide that the patient is in distress and the technician must be prepared to provide the necessary critical care. If injections need to be administered, subcutaneous sites of choice include the dorsal cervical region and lateral flank area; the intramuscular sites are the epaxial muscles that course along the caudal vertebral column or the cranial aspect of the quadriceps muscle group in the rear leg.[4]

Oral suspensions that have been flavored by a compounding pharmacy are the recommended method for administering per os medications. Other oral medication flavoring options include: strawberry jam, a small piece of banana or piña colada mix. Crushed tablets or pills can be mixed in a gel substance, e.g., Nutracal®, and placed on the fur around the mouth. Rabbits, being fastidious groomers, will readily lick their fur clean and ingest the medication.

SURGICAL AND ANESTHETIC ASSISTANCE

Once the decision has been made to perform a surgical procedure, certain equipment requirements are needed for proper surgical preparation. To aid in the intubation process, a short narrow laryngoscope and a rigid plastic catheter are needed. All other surgical equipment is similar to that used for small kittens and dogs. The recommended suture material for rabbit skin is medical skin staples. Skin staples allow for rapid closure in the thin elastic skin, and most patients are unable to remove them.

Preparation of the patient prior to surgery starts with food removal 2–4 hours prior to the procedure. Presurgical antibiotic therapy is dependent on the particular procedure being performed and/or the patient's medical history. Intravenous or intraosseous catheters can be placed prior to surgery, and also in emergency situations if fluid replacement or therapeutic agents need to be quickly assimilated. All veins that were mentioned as sites for venipuncture can be used for intravenous catheter placement, but the larger veins (e.g., cephalic and saphenous) are recommended.[4] Complications, such as venous thrombi and eventual skin sloughing of the affected area make the ear vessels a poor choice for indwelling catheter placement. If an intravenous catheter cannot be placed due to vascular complications, an intraosseous catheter should be placed in the greater trochanter of the femur. Rabbit daily fluid requirements range between 50–150 ml/kg/day and may be replaced daily, divided into 3 equal amounts, or continuously through an infusion pump.[4] If the patient does not accept the catheter, then a collar needs to be applied.

Preparation of the surgical area is important and difficult when clipping thick fine rabbit fur. In addition, the skin is thin, elastic, and easily traumatized. The clipper blade should be held flat, close to the skin, and the fur clipped at a slow, cautious speed. Regular cleaning of the clipper blade during the preparation will improve the ability of the blade to cut the fine fur.

The surgical site should be prepped after clipping to reduce the heat loss in these small animals. General recommendations to reduce heat loss are listed in Table 4-5.[10]

Table 4-5
Rabbit Surgery Preparation

1.	Warm the immediate environment with the use of circulating water blankets or heat lamps.
2.	Clip the minimum amount of hair from the body surface at and around the surgical site.
3.	Use warmed surgical scrub solution for surgical site preparation.
4.	Avoid alcohol rinses for surgical preparation, substituting warmed saline.
5.	Cover the exposed surface of the animal with a drape.
6.	Minimize the duration of surgery and anesthesia.

ANESTHESIA

When anesthetizing a rabbit, the biggest difficulty facing the technician is the intubation process. The mouth does not open widely, the distal portion of the tongue is muscular, the larynx is in the caudal oropharynx, and rabbits are predisposed to having laryngospasms.[10] Various methods of intubation can be used, other than the oral route, including nasotracheal and a blind technique using an endotracheal tube attached to a standard stethescope.[10] Most rabbit surgical procedures that require a short time period to complete may be accomplished by inducing the patient using indicated anesthetic agents and maintaining it via facemask on isoflurane inhalation anesthesia (Tables 4-6 and 4-7).

Table 4–6
Rabbit Premedication, Sedation and Chemical Restraint Agents[10]

Drug	Dose	Comment
Acepromazine	0.25–1.0 mg/kg, IM or SC*	Good for preanesthetic use and for mild tranquilization
Fentanyl-Droperidol Innovar-Vet, Mallinckrodt Veterinary, Inc, Mundelein, IL	0.13–0.22 ml/kg, IM or SC	Excellent restraint, good analgesic qualities
Xylazine	1–5 mg/kg, IM or SC	Good sedation/analgesia May produce respiratory depression and slow heart rate Reversal agent: Yohimbine (0.2 mg/kg IV)*

* (SC = subcutaneously), (IM = intramuscularly), (IV = intravenously)

HEALTH MAINTENANCE AND DISEASES

This section will review the common rabbit diseases seen in veterinary practice. An overview of etiology, treatment, and prevention will follow a brief description of the disease presentation.

GASTRIC STASIS OR "WOOL BLOCK"

As discussed earlier in this chapter, rabbits are predisposed to hairballs when fed an improper diet. Since rabbits are unable to vomit or regurgitate stomach contents, hairballs have to be digested or passed through the intestinal tract. When hairballs become too large, gastric motility is affected and the animal becomes anorectic. Treatment includes antibiotics, cisapride (0.5 mg/kg SC q8-12h) to stimulate gastric motility, and syringe feeding the patient. A recommended recipe for syringe feeding

Table 4-7

Rabbit Injectable Anesthetic Agents[10]

Drug	Dose	Comment
Diazepam/Ketamine	Diazepam (0.5 mg/kg) and Ketamine (10–20 mg/kg) IV	Good for sedation and adjunct to supplemental inhalation anesthesia
Tiletamine-Zolazepam	5–25 mg/kg IM	Light sedation and general anesthesia
		High dose may cause severe depression, slow recovery, and possible nephrotoxicity
Xylazine/Ketamine	1. Xylazine (3–5 mg/kg) and Ketamine (20–40 mg/kg) IM	Good for some surgical procedures
	2. Xylazine (3 mg/kg) and Ketamine (10 mg/kg) intranasal	Remember Xylazine may cause respiratory depression and hypotension
		Intranasal administration good for short-term anesthesia

is: one cup rabbit pellets, one 8 oz. can Ensure®, and one 8 oz. container of fruit yogurt; blend and feed via syringe. If obese rabbits are not fed and subsequently develop a negative energy balance, hepatic lipidosis will occur. Prevention of the disease is the best method of treatment. Prevention of hairballs in rabbits is initiated through owner education on proper dietary requirements.

GASTROENTERITIS

Antibiotics may cause a fatal gastrointestinal bacterial overgrowth if administered to rabbits. **Never use the following unless they are the absolute last resort for treatment: clindamycin, amoxicillin and derivatives, ampicillin, penicillin, cephalosporins, and erythromycin.** Always make sure that the drug being given is appropriate to use in rabbits. Treatment of gastroenteritis is similar to other pets, i.e., maintaining hydration status, identification of the causative agent, and proper treatment. *E. coli*, *Clostridium piliforme*, *Salmonella* spp., and *Pseudomonas* spp. are common bacterial organisms that cause gastroenteritis.

PASTEURELLA MULTOCIDA "SNUFFLES"

This is the most common disease affecting pet rabbits. *Pasteurella multocida* can infect all major body systems (especially the respiratory system) and major organs; and it can cause subcutaneous abscesses (Figure 4-10). Another common presentation is a head tilt, which is often the result of an internal ear infection associated with *P. multocida* (Figure 4-11). This bacterium can survive within a rabbit host for years

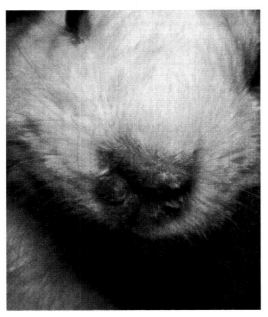

Figure 4-10 Nasal discharge due to *Pasteurella multocida* infection (snuffles).

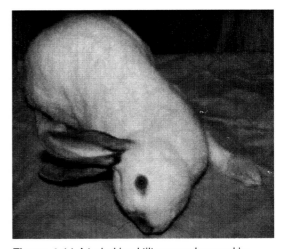

Figure 4-11 A typical head tilt commonly caused by *Pasteurella multocida (otitis media).*

without causing any overt disease signs. During this period, shedding can take place, which can then infect any rabbit that comes into contact with the infected animal. Treatment has improved with Baytril® enrofloxacin 5–10 mg/kg orally q14 days. There is no guarantee that the treatment will rid the patient of the infection, but treatment is usually successful in reducing the disease signs associated with the infection. The bacterial organism is transmitted through direct contact, fomites, and sexual intercourse—but usually gains entry into the host through the nares or wounds. Culture of the respiratory system, through the nares, is usually the best way to confirm a diagnosis, but response to treatment of this pervasive disease precludes diagnostic testing. The best prevention with this disease is client education and the purchase of rabbits from reputable breeders that have a *P. multocida*-free herd.

MALOCCLUSION

Overgrowth of the incisors and/or the cheek teeth is a problem often affecting pet rabbits (Figure 4-12). Malocclusion of the teeth may present as a rabbit not being able to chew

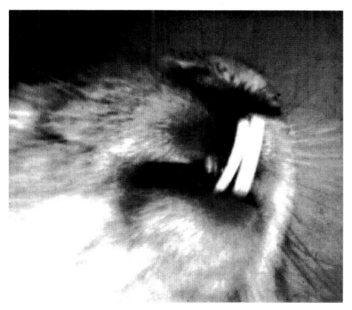

and hold the food in its mouth or excessive drooling around the edges of the mouth. A complete oral examination is required for each patient. The incisors may be examined by using a tongue depressor and moving the lips to observe the teeth. If maloccluded, the upper incisors grow behind the bottom incisors. Genetics and traumatic injury appear to be the main sources of this disease. The cheek teeth are best examined using an

Figure 4-12 Incisor overgrowth due to malocclusion. This condition requires a routine trimming schedule to maintain normal eating habits and health.

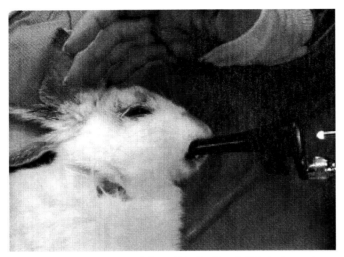

Figure 4-13 Otoscope examining rabbit cheek teeth. This instrument needs to be used to properly examine the cheek teeth because of the small oral cavity.

otoscope (Figure 4-13). The teeth can be trimmed using small clippers and the cheek teeth floated, using small rabbit floats and specula for exposure in the small oral cavity (Figure 4-14). Affected patients never "grow out" of this problem and have to be treated on a regular basis. Removal of the overgrown teeth is not recommended, unless there is a complicating abscess at the base of the tooth.

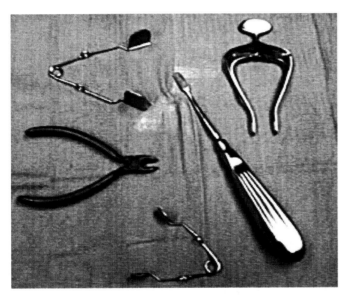

Figure 4-14 Specific dental instruments used to treat rabbit malocclusion problems.

"SORE HOCKS" OR ULCERATIVE PODODERMATITIS

An infection of the plantar surface of the hock is called ulcerative pododermatitis. This condition is usually the result of poor husbandry practices by the owner. Once the hock area ulcerates because of improper flooring, secondary bacterial infections infiltrate the wound. This is a very difficult disease to treat, and owner understanding and compliance are essential for a successful outcome. The environment needs to be cleaned, and the wounds must be cleaned and bandaged.

ZOONOTIC DISEASES

There are not many cases of diseases being transmitted from rabbits to their human caretakers. Although not common, disease transmission can and does occur. Common bacterial pathogens that may be transferred include *Salmonella* spp., *Pasteurella multocida,* and bacteria through scratches or bites. Dermatophyte (ringworm) infections can cause dry crusty lesions on rabbits that exhibit hair loss. The most common dermatophyte isolated in pet rabbits is *Trichophyton mentagrophytes*, which is extremely zoonotic to children and older adults.

REFERENCES

1. Donnelly, T.M. "Basic Anatomy, Physiology and Husbandry." In Hillyer, E.V. and Quesenberry, K.E. eds., *Ferrets, Rabbits and Rodents: Clinical Medicine and Surgery.* Philadelphia: W.B. Saunders, 1997: 147–59.

2. Cheeke, P.R. *Rabbit Feeding and Nutrition.* Orlando, Florida: Academic Press, 1987: 15–33.

3. Brooks, D. "Nutrition and Gastrointestinal Physiology." In Hillyer, E.V. and Quesenberry, K.E., eds. *Ferrets, Rabbits and Rodents: Clinical Medicine and Surgery.* Philadelphia: W.B. Saunders, 1997: 169–75.

4. Mader, D.R. "Basic Approach to Veterinary Care" In Hillyer, E.V. and Quesenberry, K.E. eds., *Ferrets, Rabbits and Rodents. Clinical Medicine and Surgery.* Philadelphia: W.B. Saunders, 1997: 161–66.

5. Benson, K.G. and Paul-Murphy, J. "Clinical Pathology of the Domestic Rabbit." In Rupley, A.E. and Reavill, D.R. eds., *The Vet Clinics of North America, Exotic Animal Practice, Clinical Pathology and Sample Collection.* Philadelphia: W.B. Saunders, 1999: 2(3)(Sep): 539–51.

6. Johnson-Delaney, C.A. and Harrison, L.R. *Rabbits, Exotic Companion Medicine Handbook for Veterinarians*. Lake Worth, Florida: Wingers Publishing, 1996: 9–10

7. Harkness, J.E. and Wagner, J.E. *The Biology and Medicine of Rabbits and Rodents*. 3rd ed., Lea & Febiger, 1989.

8. Harkness, J.E. and Wagner, J.E. *The Biology and Medicine of Rabbits and Rodents*. 4th ed., Lea & Febiger, 1995.

9. Quesenberry, K.E. "Rabbits." In Birchard, S.J., Sherding, R.G. eds., *Saunders Manual of Small Animal Practice*. Philadelphia: WB Saunders, 1994: 1345–7.

10. Hillyer, E.V. "Dermatologic Diseases" In Hillyer, E.V. and Quesenberry, K.E. eds., *Ferrets, Rabbits and Rodents: Clinical Medicine and Surgery*. Philadelphia: W.B. Saunders, 1997: 215–17.

11. Mason, D.E. "Anesthesia, Analgesia and Sedation for Small Mammals." In Hillyer, E.V. and Quesenberry, K.E. eds., *Ferrets, Rabbits and Rodents: Clinical Medicine and Surgery*. Philadelphia: W.B. Saunders, 1997: 378–91.

CHAPTER 5

RODENTS

GUINEA PIGS

INTRODUCTION

Guinea pigs (*Cavia porcellus*) are native to the Andean highlands of north-central and northwestern South America.[1] There are three main breeds that are maintained as companion animals: 1) the English or common, which is characterized with short, straight, fine hair; 2) the Abyssinian with rough, wiry hair in rosettes or whorls; and 3) the Peruvian with long, straight, silky hair (Figures 5-1A, 5-1B, and 5-1C). Of all rodent species, guinea pigs may be the best choice for pets. They are usually nonaggressive, rarely bite, enjoy being held, and are long-lived in comparison to many other rodents.

With the advent of commercial guinea pig diets and supplies by a large number of companies, it has never been easier to properly care for these rodents. Cavies (a common name for guinea pigs) belong to a group of animals that requires an external source of vitamin C. Often, the vitamin C is incorporated into the diet, but if the diet is deficient in the daily requirement of this essential vitamin, supplementation must be provided in the water or on the food. Vitamin C deficiency is one of the most common health problems treated by veterinarians. This information, along with basic dietary

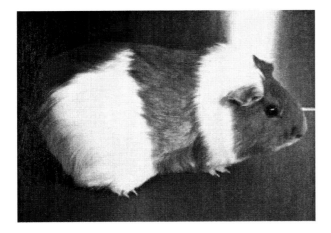

suggestions and husbandry techniques, should be provided to the owner during the cavy's first veterinary examination. To determine the health status of the patient and to answer basic questions, a technician should be familiar with baseline guinea pig physiologic information (Table 5-1).

Figure 5-1A The English, or common, is one of the types of guinea pigs maintained as pets.

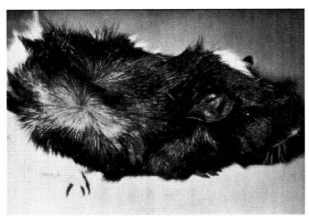

Figure 5-1B Abyssinian guinea pigs are commonly kept as companion animals.

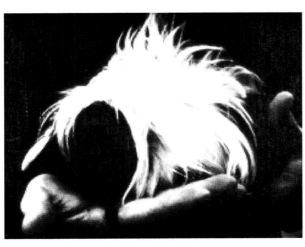

Figure 5-1C Peruvian guinea pigs have long straight, silky hair.

Table 5-1
Guinea Pig Basic Information[2]

Body weight	Adult male	900–1200 g
	Adult female	750–900 g
	Birth weight	60–110 g
Temperature, pulse and respiration	Rectal body temperature	101.5–103°F
	Normal heart rate	230–380 beats/minute
	Normal respiratory rate	42–104 breaths/minute
Amounts of food and water	Daily food consumption	6g/100 g body weight/day
	Daily water consumption	10 ml/100 g body weight/day
Age at onset of puberty and breeding initiation	Puberty males	9–10 weeks
	Puberty females	6 weeks
	Breeding initiation males	3–4 months
	Breeding initiation females	2–3 months
Female reproductive cycle	Estrous cycle	15–17 days
	Estrus duration	1–16 hours (average 8 hours)
	Gestation length	59–72 days
	Litter size	3–4 average

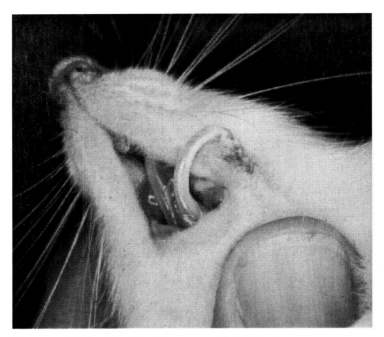

Figure 5-2 Teeth malocclusion is an overgrowth of the incisors.

As with other animals in the order Rodentia, guinea pigs have open-rooted teeth. Open-rooted teeth continuously grow; thus, they need a normal occlusive surface to wear properly and prevent overgrowth. It is common in cavies to have malocclusion of the cheek teeth, which causes enamel projections to rub against the tongue surface (Figure "5-2). This condition is commonly called "slobbers" by guinea pig owners because the irritation promotes salivation and anorexia.

HUSBANDRY

ENVIRONMENTAL CONCERNS

Guinea pigs are commonly maintained in indoor cages. The general environment of the house will usually provide an adequate temperature range to maintain proper health and comfort. These animals are native to the Andean mountain range and are more sensitive to warmer temperatures than to cooler ones. Temperatures above 80–85°F may cause heat-related deaths.[1]

A guinea pig enclosure should have one cubic foot of space per adult and be made out of wire mesh (0.5–1.5" spacing). Breeders should have twice the recommended adult floor space.[2] The cage should have an open top with sides at least 10" high and should also have a hiding box to provide security when needed.[1] Cavies are very susceptible to infectious pododermatitis, or "bumblefoot." A solid floor is preferred over a wire mesh floor to prevent bumblefoot and protect against limb and nail trauma. Other pets that may harm guinea pigs, such as dogs and cats, should be kept in an area that will prevent an attack and exposure to *Bordetella* spp. bacteria.

As with all rodents and pocket pets, bedding must be changed on a regular basis because fecal, urine, food, and water soil the environment. Hardwood shavings, composite recycled paper materials, pellets, and shredded paper may be used as bedding material. Guinea pigs are also susceptible to submandibular abscesses, commonly called "lumps." These abscesses are caused by hay, straw, or woodchips that are eaten and puncture the gingival surface—seeding bacteria within the oral cavity. The bacterial infection migrates into the submandibular/cervical area forming large abscesses. If a patient presents with these abscesses, the diet should be reviewed in order to help identify and eliminate the initiating cause of the problem.

NUTRITION

A commercial guinea pig feed (20% crude protein and 16% fiber) is the best basic diet, along with free choice of timothy hay.[2] Many companies manufacture guinea pig kibble, pellets, or biscuits, and this should be the base diet. Please discourage use of any rodent diet that contains seed. The dietary source should be fresh and supplemented with ascorbic acid (vitamin C). If the diet is not fresh (within 30 days of milling date), there is a possibility that the vitamin content has degraded and is not adequate for the pet's daily requirements. Supplemental vitamin C will aid in the cavy's general health; they require 7–10 mg/kg/day and, if pregnant, 20–30 mg/kg/day.[1] Kale, cabbage, and oranges are very good dietary sources of vitamin C. Tang®, an instant orange drink, can be mixed into the sipper bottle water and this will provide additional vitamin C. Any vitamin C supplement that is added to the water must be reformulated and changed daily because the half-life is only 24 hours in glass bottles of clean water.[1] Timothy hay, alfalfa cubes, small amounts of green vegetables, and apples are all treats that these animals eat on a regular basis.[2] Treats should be limited to 1–2 tablespoons over a 24-hour period with the bulk of the dietary requirements coming from guinea pig chow.[2] Feeders and sipper tubes should be suspended on the side of the cage to prevent fecal contamination and dumping of the contents on the cage floor.

HISTORY

The same questions used to obtain a history for other small rodents and pocket pets can be used for the guinea pig patient. The history and physical examination sections in the following rodent and pocket pet sections will not be repeated. It is recommended that this section be referred to when examining these animals.

The same basic background information is required for guinea pigs as for other animals that are examined at the veterinary clinic. How long the animal has been owned, where it was acquired, how often it is handled, and the character of the feces and urine are a few of the questions that should be asked for background information. Husbandry questions include: where the animal is housed; whether it is allowed to roam unobserved in the house; cage location, type, size, material, substrate, furniture, toys, how often the cage is cleaned and the disinfectant that is used. When investigating the diet, it is important to ask if pellets are fed, how much, and also what the animal is actually eating. Supplemental offerings and frequency of feeding are very important data for the case work-up. To round out the nutrition section, the technician should find out about the water supply, how often the water is changed, and how much the animal drinks on a daily basis.

Since there are transmissible diseases between animals, the final questions should center on other pets in the household—if new animals have been added to the family or if the animals are housed together. Finally, a description of any previous problems and a complete chronological description of the presenting problem are needed to complete the history form.

RESTRAINT

Guinea pigs should be restrained by grabbing the animal around the shoulders with one hand, lifting the animal up, and supporting the rear with the other hand (Figure 5-3). The handler must be careful not to squeeze too hard with the hand around the neck and chest. If too much pressure is placed on the guinea pig's thoracic region, respiratory compromise may occur. To prevent possible respiratory distress, the handler should place the hand around the neck from the ventral aspect of the animal, while supporting the rear legs with the other hand.

PHYSICAL EXAMINATION

Prior to restraint, an observation should be made about the attitude, activity, and posture of the animal. The next step is to weigh the guinea pig in a basket on a digital gram scale. If possible, temperature, respiration, and pulse should be measured and any abnormalities in rate and/or character noted. The physical examination starts at the head, looking for any abnormalities. Eyes, ears, and nares are observed, looking for discharge or inflammation. The oral cavity is difficult to examine in guinea pigs because of the small opening and tendency for the buccal mucosa to encroach toward the middle of the mouth. A small rabbit specula or an otoscope may be used to examine the oral cavity and teeth. Mucous membranes help determine hydration status using capillary refill time and moisture. Body condition and abdominal palpation findings are important information that should be obtained.

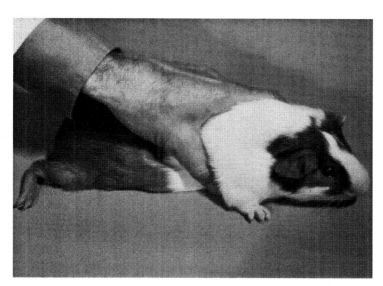

Figure 5-3 Proper holding position. Although friendly, guinea pigs need to be properly held for adequate physical examination.

Lymph nodes and limbs are palpated prior to checking the nails and plantar surface of each foot. The patient should have a normal posture, be aware of its surroundings, and move properly. Any problems should be noted in the record. Finally, a dermatological exam considers hair coat quality, alopecia, external parasites, or any skin abnormalities. All abnormal findings are written in the record for case review, differential diagnosis determination, diagnostic testing, and treatment considerations.

DIAGNOSTIC SAMPLING

BLOOD COLLECTION

In guinea pigs and other pocket pets, blood collection can be quite difficult. Approximately 0.5–0.7 ml/100 grams of body weight can be safely removed from a non-anemic, healthy guinea pig.[3] The easiest veins to see are the lateral saphenous and cephalic, but they are very small and collapse easily. The fur should be clipped over the vein from which the blood will be taken and the surfaced prepared with alcohol. A small 25- or 26-gauge needle, usually placed on a 3-cc syringe, is recommended to collect the blood. The short jugular vein may be used, but it is difficult to find, and the cranial vena cava may lead to bleeding complications (if used in cavies). The position to collect from the jugular vein is similar to the technique used in cats. Reference ranges for complete blood counts and serum chemistry panels are listed in Tables 5-2 and 5-3.[3]

Table 5-2
Guinea Pig Complete Blood Count Reference Ranges

Erythrocytes	$3.2–8.0 \times 10^6/\mu l$
Hematocrit	32–50%
Hemoglobin	10–17 g/dl
Leukocytes	$5.5–17.5 \times 10^3/\mu l$
Neutrophils	22–48%
Lymphocytes	39–72%
Eosinophils	0–7%
Monocytes	1–10%
Basophils	0–2.7%
Platelets	$260–740 \times 10^3/\mu l$
Serum protein	4.2–6.8 g/dl
Albumin	2.1–3.9 g/dl
Globulin	1.7–2.6 g/dl

Table 5-3
Guinea Pig Serum Biochemistry Reference Ranges

Serum glucose	60–125 mg/dl
Blood urea nitrogen	9.0–31.5 mg/dl
Creatinine	0.6–2.2 mg/dl
Total bilirubin	0–0.9 mg/dl
Cholesterol	16–43 mg/dl
Serum calcium	8.2–12.0 mg/dl
Serum phosphorus	3.0–7.6 mg/dl
Alkaline phosphatase	55–108 U/L
Alanine aminotransferase (ALT)	25–59 U/L
Aspartate aminotransferase (AST)	26–68 U/L

BONE MARROW ASPIRATION

Marrow samples may be obtained from the ilium, tibia, sternum, femur, or the bones of the proximal one-third of the tail.[4] Preparation of the samples is consistent with that of other mammalian patients.

URINE COLLECTION

When the patient is hospitalized, a standard rodent cage (without substrate) can be used to collect urine and feces. The sample can also be collected by placing a small rodent in an unsealed Zip-lock® bag, which will often cause the animal to urinate. For guinea pigs and larger pocket pets, a standard cystocentesis procedure can be used to collect urine directly from the bladder.

MICROBIOLOGY AND RADIOLOGY

As mentioned earlier, guinea pigs are susceptible to *Bordetella bronchiseptica* and *Streptococcus pneumonia* respiratory bacterial infections. It is best to prevent these respiratory infections by separating other pets (dogs, cats, and rabbits) from the guinea pigs. *Staphylococcus aureus* is the major causative agent found in infectious pododermatitis lesions. *Streptococcus zooepidemicus* and *Streptobacillus moniliformis* are common isolates of infections affecting the cervical lymph nodes commonly called "lumps." Routine culture techniques should be used to isolate and identify the bacterial organism causing a disease.

Radiology techniques for guinea pigs and other pocket pets are similar to those used on rabbits. **Please refer to the rabbit chapter for radiology techniques needed for guinea pigs and pocket pets.**

PARASITOLOGY

Ectoparasites

Guinea pigs can be infested by mites, lice, and fleas. The most significant ectoparasite is the sarcoptic mite, *Trixacarus caviae*.[3] Guinea pigs infested with *T. caviae* have intense itching episodes that result in hair loss and skin lesions, primarily involving the thighs and back.[3] Treatment of guinea pigs diagnosed with *T. caviae* is difficult because the environment and animal must be treated at the same time. The enclosure should be cleaned at least twice a week during the treatment period, and all toys and bedding material should be removed. It is important to discuss the zoonotic potential of *T. caviae* with the owner. During the treatment phase, the owner should wear latex gloves, and exposure to other family members and pets should be limited during the recovery period. Once the guinea pig has been treated, and no mites remain, new toys should be purchased.

Lice and mites, including *T. caviae,* can be treated with ivermectin (Ivomec, Merck & Co., Inc, West Point, PA, 0.5 mg/kg, SC and repeat in 10 days). Unfortunately, *T. caviae* and other guinea pig parasites are becoming resistant to ivermectin treatment alone, so 4 to 5 treatments of ivermectin (10 days apart) are needed, with the owner cleaning the environment twice a week. To aid in treatment of difficult mite and lice infestations, lime sulfur dip (2.5% solution, apply once per week for 4–6 weeks) is also prescribed as an adjunct therapy. The combined treatment protocol usually works well.

Guinea pigs are exposed to ectoparasites through direct contact. Most of the animals that are affected are recent purchases from a pet store. If fleas are a problem, a pyrethrin-based cat flea powder is effective, especially after the environment is treated and the patient has been bathed.

Internal Parasites

There are not many internal parasites of consequence that are commonly diagnosed in pet guinea pigs. *Cryptosporidium wrairi* is a protozoal diarrhea that infects the small intestine and can cause death.[5] Clinical signs are consistent with other gastrointestinal illnesses, including diarrhea, anorexia, and weight loss. As mentioned previously, this infection is rare, but possibly zoonotic. There is no effective treatment for guinea pigs with this disease.

THERAPEUTICS

This section will include the therapeutic issues for all small mammals and pocket pets. The size of these patients contributes to the difficulty in properly administering therapeutic medication. The scruff of the neck or caudal flank are the subcutaneous sites that may be utilized to administer medication and/or fluids.[7] The semitendinosus, triceps, and/or epaxial muscles are commonly used for intramuscular injections, while intraperitoneal injections are used in extremely small species.[7] On larger rodents and pocket pets, intravenous injections can be given in the cephalic, saphenous, or jugular vein.[7] Intraosseous catheters are much easier to administer in these small animals than intravenous catheters. The tibial plateau or the greater trochanter are the sites of choice for intraosseous catheter placement in pocket pets.[7]

Although many methods may be used to administer medication in small mammals, oral treatment (using a dropper or tuberculin syringe) is the easiest and least stressful to the patient. Medication can be added to the food or water, but often the patient is anorexic, which means that the medicated food/water is not palatable. Hence, the patient does not self-treat.

SURGICAL AND ANESTHETIC ASSISTANCE

Inducing and maintaining guinea pigs, other small rodents, and pocket pets under anesthesia can be very challenging. With the widespread use of isoflurane anesthesia in small animal practices, the previous problems associated with injection, methoxyflurane, and halothane anesthetic agents have been overcome. There are still concerns and differences in anesthetic protocol because of these animals' small size, but in general, isoflurane anesthesia is a safe agent when used on a relatively healthy surgical candidate.

An induction chamber is used to induce the patients and then they are maintained under gas anesthesia using a facemask (Figure 5-4). While it may be possible to intubate a larger rodent or pocket pet, it is very difficult under most conditions.[8]

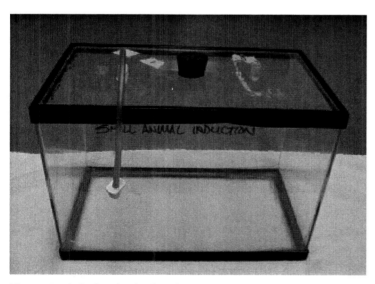

Figure 5-4 Induction chamber for guinea pigs or other small rodents.

Guinea pigs have a tendency to regurgitate gastric contents when under general anesthesia; therefore, it is recommended to fast these animals at least 2–4 hours prior to surgery.[8] To guard against aspiration of stomach contents in a patient that is not intubated, place the head and neck in a position slightly higher than the body.

Table 5-4 provides guidelines for surgical preparation and assistance in surgical procedures on small exotic animals.[9]

Table 5-4
Basic Surgery Guidelines for Rodents and Pocket Pets[9]

1. Obtain accurate body weight
2. Know the appropriate preoperative fasting interval
3. Properly dose and administer medication
4. Minimize stress through premedication or minimal handling
5. Administer oxygen when using only injection anesthesia
6. Prevent hypothermia by using external heat sources
7. Provide fluid therapy and maintain hemostasis during surgery

Table 5–5
Premedication and Sedation Drug Doses for Rodents[9]

All doses are mg/kg and should be given IM or SC

Drug	Guinea Pig	Rat	Mouse	Hamster	Gerbil
Acepromazine	0.5–1.5	0.5–2.5	0.5–2.5	0.5–5	0
Diazepam	1–5	3–5	3–5	3–5	3–5
Midazolam	1–2	1–2	1–2	1–2	1–2
Xylazine*	5–10	10–15	10–15	8–10	5–10
Atropine	0.05	0.05	0.05	0.05	0.05

* Xylazine has a reversal agent – Yohimine (0.2 mg/kg IV)

Premedication and sedation doses for rodents are listed in Table 5-5. If the surgeon wants to perform the procedure under injectable general anesthesia, the doses are listed in Table 5-6. Analgesia is important for patient recovery and should be administered prior to, during, and after surgery—depending on the case presentation and procedure being performed. In Table 5-7, analgesic drug doses are listed for small animals.

Table 5-6
Injectable Anesthesia in Rodents[9]

All doses are mg/kg and should be given IM				
Drug	**Guinea Pig**	**Rat**	**Mouse**	**Hamster**	**Gerbil**
Acepromazine/ Ketamine	0.5–1.0 20–50	2.5–5.0 50–150	2.5–5.0 50–150	2.5–5.0 50–150	0
Xylazine/ Ketamine	3–5 20–40	5 90	5–10 50–200	5–10 50–150	2–3 50–70
Diazepam/ Ketamine	3–5 20–40	3–5 40–100	3–5 40–150	5 40–150	3–5 40–150
Tiletamine-Zolazepam	20–40	50–80	50–80	50–80	50–80

Table 5–7
Analgesic Dosages for Rodents

All dosages are mg/kg and should be given SC or IM				
Drug	**Guinea Pig**	**Rat**	**Mouse**	**Gerbil**	**Hamster**
Butorphanol	2 (q2–4h)	2 (q2–4h)	1–5 (q2–4h)	1–5 (q2–4h)	1–5 (q2–4h)
Buprenorphine	0.005 (q8–12h)	0.05–0.1 (q8–12h)	0.05–0.1 (q8–12h)	0.05–0.1 (q8–12h)	0.05–0.1 (q8–12h)

DISEASES

This section will review the common guinea pig diseases seen in veterinary practice. An overview of etiology, treatment, and prevention will follow a brief description of the disease presentation.

SCURVY

Guinea pigs lack the ability to endogenously synthesize ascorbic acid. Therefore, to maintain proper health, it is essential that a dietary supplement of vitamin C be provided. Common signs associated with vitamin C deficiency include hemorrhage in the joints and gingiva, malocclusion, rough hair-coat, alopecia, anorexia, lameness, and bruxism. The daily vitamin C supplementation for guinea pigs is 15–25 mg/day and pregnant animals 30 mg/day.[6] Vitamin C can be ingested in the food and water or on the food as a supplement. Fresh cabbage, kale, or oranges provide sources of supplemental vitamin C.[6]

"BUMBLEFOOT"

Bumblefoot, or infectious pododermatitis, is usually the result of foot pad trauma progressing into a chronic *Staphylococcus aureus* infection.[6] The initiating cause of many bumblefoot infections is inadequate caging substrate, particularly wire-bottom cages and abrasive bedding material. Owners must be informed of the guarded prognosis in resolving these foot infections. Surgical debridement, topical and systemic antibiotic treatment, and bandaging of the affected feet are required to improve the chances of recovery. To prevent recurrence, the owner should change the substrate and floor of the cage into a solid floor with nonabrasive bedding.

"LUMPS"

Lumps is a common term given to a disease of the cervical lymph nodes that results in abscessation due to a *Streptococcus zooepidemicus* infection. *S. zooepidemicus* is part of the normal flora of guinea pig conjunctival and nasal mucosa.[6] Once the oral mucosa is compromised, usually by poor quality hay, the bacteria travel through the blood stream into the cervical lymph nodes. Complete surgical excision of the affected lymph nodes is recommended for treating the disease. The owner should be informed of the disease process and measures taken to prevent recurrence, including stress reduction and a quality diet.

MALOCCLUSION

Guinea pigs have open-rooted incisors, premolars, and molars. Open-rooted teeth grow continuously and, if the teeth are not properly aligned, malocclusion will occur—resulting in overgrowth of the affected teeth. All of the teeth previously mentioned can become overgrown, resulting in anorexia and hypersalivation. The teeth should be trimmed on a regular basis to prevent the physical inability to eat and trauma to the tongue and buccal surface. General anesthesia is recommended for trimming of the molars and premolars, while the incisors can be trimmed using regular restraint. Vitamin C deficiency has been implicated as a possible contributor to the disease process due to the breakdown of collagen formation in the tooth socket, causing instability that leads to malocclusion.

ANTIBIOTIC-ASSOCIATED ENTEROTOXEMIA

When treating guinea pigs with antibiotics, it must be remembered that their normal gastrointestinal flora are predominantly Gram-positive organisms.[6] Classes of drugs that include penicillin and aminoglycosides will kill the normal gastrointestinal flora causing an overgrowth of *Clostridium difficile*.[6] **Never prescribe antibiotics for a guinea pig patient unless there is a reference for its use in this species.** Other antibiotics that are recommended for use in guinea pigs should be monitored during the treatment period. If there is any evidence of the patient becoming anorexic or having diarrhea, the medication should be discontinued and the patient rechecked for drug induced gastroenteritis.

ZOONOTIC DISEASES

There are not many zoonotic diseases associated with guinea pigs. The zoonotic diseases that may cause problems are rarely transmitted to human caretakers. *Trixacarus caviae* or the guinea pig sarcoptic mite may be the most problematic. When treating a mite infestation, owners should take precautions against exposure.

Guinea pig dermatophyte, or "ringworm" infections, can be transmitted to humans. Dermatophyte infections, particularly *Trichophyton mentagrophytes,* do not commonly affect guinea pigs; but if diagnosed, environmental cleaning and patient treatment is required to resolve the disease condition. Again, owners should be instructed to use caution to prevent exposure and possible contamination.

Small Pet Rodents:
Hamsters, Gerbils, Rats, and Mice

INTRODUCTION

The small pet rodent information will be compiled into one section. Some data is listed in other areas of the text, and the reader will be referred to that specific section. The four common small rodent species maintained as pets—hamsters, gerbils, rats, and mice—will be covered separately within this section. There are many similarities in care, husbandry, diagnostic testing, and treatment for these animals. There will be an emphasis on the differences between the species and a conscious effort to restrict redundant information.

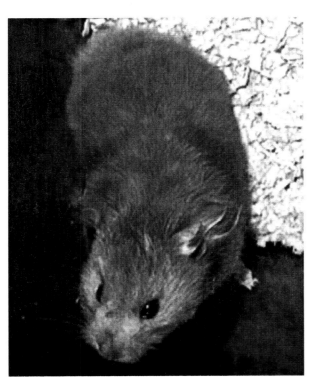

Figure 5-5 The teddy bear hamster is a common type of pet hamster.

HAMSTERS

The golden or Syrian hamster *(Mesocricetus auratus)* is a very popular pet due to its small size and "cute" appearance, especially the Teddy Bear (Figure 5-5). The golden hamster is the most popular pet species of hamsters, but there are also Chinese, European, Hungarian, and Siberian dwarf hamsters (Figure 5-6). Although cute and small, these small rodents can be territorial and aggressive, and they can bite their owners. Reduction of the animal's natural aggressive personality is usually achieved through routine handling. To reduce fighting between pet hamsters, animals should be housed in separate cages. All gender combinations will fight or succumb

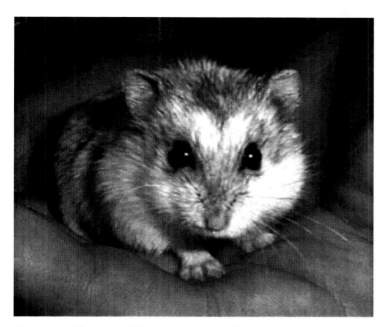

Figure 5-6 Siberian dwarf hamsters are also popular pets.

to immunosuppression initiated by psychological stress levels due to a dominant animal within the environment. Females that have given birth will often cannibalize their young if disturbed.

Hamsters are nocturnal animals and like to exercise during the night. If the exercise wheel is not oiled, the squeaking apparatus may disturb the owner. These animals are notorious for escaping their enclosure. The owner must understand the importance of purchasing an escape-proof cage with an appropriate screen top that can be fastened securely.

Veterinary technicians need to be aware of a few anatomical differences found in hamsters. (See the baseline hamster physical information listed in Table 5-8. [1]) The most prominent are the large cheek pouches that can store large pellets, seed, or bedding material. It is very common for hamsters to have full cheek pouches, which deforms the face, but this is a normal behavior pattern for these animals. Male hamsters have two small, symmetrical black spots on the lateral flank region of the body. These are lateral flank sebaceous glands. The glands are testosterone dependent and are better developed in males than females.[2] The only open-rooted teeth in small rodents, including hamsters, are the incisors.

To properly sex hamsters, rats, mice, and gerbils, the distance from the anus to the genital opening is measured. This distance in males is twice that of female animals.[2] Females have three openings in this area (urinary, genital, and anal), while males have two openings (urogenital and anal).[2]

Table 5-8
Hamster Basic Information[1]

Body weight	Adult male	85–130 grams
	Adult female	95–150 grams
	Birth weight	2 grams
Temperature, pulse and respiration	Rectal body temperature	99–101°F
	Normal heart rate	25–500 beats/minute
	Normal respiratory rate	35–135 breaths/minute
Amounts of food and water	Daily food consumption	>15 g/100 g body weight/day
	Daily water consumption	>20 ml/100 g body weight/day
Age at onset of puberty and breeding initiation	Puberty males	45–75 days
	Breeding initiation males	10–14 weeks
	Breeding initiation females	6–10 weeks
Female reproductive cycle	Estrous cycle	4 days (polyestrous)
	Gestation length	15–18 days
	Litter size	5–9 average

HUSBANDRY

ENVIRONMENTAL CONCERNS

As discussed previously, hamsters commonly chew their way out of enclosures. It is important that the housing be "hamster-proof" or the animal may escape into the house. If a hamster does escape, the best way to capture it is to place food in the center of the room. Once it has been determined in which room the animal is hiding, the room should be sealed. Since hamsters are nocturnal animals, capturing them at night—in a dark room, with a flashlight—may work best. This technique will work for the capture of other small rodents and pocket pets.

The recommended cage size for hamsters, mice, and gerbils is 20" x 20" x 6–10" high.[1] The cage should provide enough room for the animal to exercise and should contain an exercise wheel and a hiding box. For proper ventilation, a screen top is recommended. Hardwood shaving or shredded papers are the primary substrate choices for rodent cages, with cleaning occurring 1 to 2 times a week. If the plastic tube housing systems are used, a routine cleaning of the sections using hot water and a mild detergent is called for. Ventilation is essential in all small rodent housing to prevent irritation of the respiratory tract from the ammonia vapors generated by urine.

NUTRITION

The nutritional requirements for most small rodents are the same. There are a number of commercial hamster/rodent pellets available. The formulas that contain at least 16% protein and 8% fiber provide for optimum health.[1,2] The owner should be informed that any seed-based rodent diet is unacceptable for health maintenance. Treats may be offered in the form of nuts, raisins, apple, and greens, at no more than 1/2 teaspoon per 24 hours.[1]

Sipper bottles and small food containers that fit on the side of the enclosure reduce spillage and urinary/fecal contamination. Water and feed containers should be cleaned daily and replenished with fresh contents.

HISTORY

(See guinea pig section.)

RESTRAINT

Hamsters and small rodents can be restrained by pinching the skin on the scruff of the neck. It is important to get a tight hold of the skin to prevent escape or injury. Hamsters' eyes may prolapse with a tight grip, but gentle pressure on the globe, pushing into the orbit, usually resolves the problem.

PHYSICAL EXAMINATION

(See guinea pig section.)

DIAGNOSTIC SAMPLING

BLOOD COLLECTION

Although hamsters, gerbils, and rats are very small animals, blood must be collected and tested for diagnostic purposes. Clipping the hair and disinfecting the topical skin surface will properly prepare the blood collection sites. General anesthesia is a consideration whenever blood is being collected for diagnostic testing in these small animals. Usually, inducing the animals in a closed chamber and maintaining the patients in a mask will allow the technician plenty of time to collect the blood sample. Table 5-9 describes the technique used for retro-orbital blood collection in small rodents (Figure 5-7).

On smaller rodents, the saphenous vein or lateral vein of the tarsus may be used for multiple blood collections without the use of anesthesia. The patient must be properly immobilized in a restraint tube (35-cc syringe) with the leg extended and the skin held tight on the medial aspect of the thigh using the thumb and forefinger. The taut skin on the lateral aspect of the thigh allows exposure of the saphenous vein. A 23-gauge needle is used to puncture the vein, and blood is collected in a microhematocrit tube as it flows from the vessel.[3]

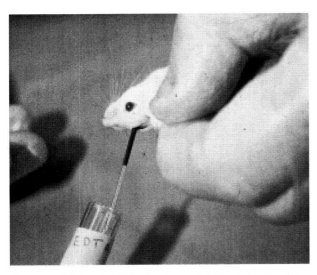

Figure 5-7 Retro-orbital bleeding is a common technique used to obtain blood samples from rodents.

The jugular vein and ear vessel may be used in larger rodents and pocket pets for blood collection. To collect blood from the jugular vein, a 3-cc syringe and 25-gauge needle are needed, while a microhematocrit tube is used for the ear vessel. Blood samples obtained from nail and ear clips are not considered appropriate diagnostic samples. Cardiac puncture is only recommended on terminal cases, when the animal is maintained under general anesthesia, because of possible complications involving the lungs and heart vessels. Reference ranges for complete blood counts and serum chemistry panels are listed in Tables 5-10 and 5-11.[1]

BONE MARROW ASPIRATION AND URINE COLLECTION

(See guinea pig section.)

FECAL EXAMINATION AND ANAL TAPE TEST

Routine fecal parasite evaluations should be performed on small rodents when presented for a health examination or an abnormal stool. Common protozoal organisms that can be detected using a direct fecal examination include *Giardia* spp., cryptosporidiosis,

Table 5-9
Retro-orbital Blood Collection[3]

1. Stabilize head at base of skull and point of jaw.
2. Occlusion of the jugular vein may distend the venous plexus.
3. Retract the dorsal lid of the eye with the index finger.
4. Collection
   a) Hamsters – a microcapillary tube or small-bore Pasteur pipette is inserted midway along the superior border of the eye and advanced to the plexus located posterior to the globe.[4]
   b) Mice and Gerbils – a microcapillary tube or small-bore Pasteur pipette is inserted at the medial canthus.
   c) Rats – the middorsal approach, similar to the hamster approach, is considered the most direct access to the dorsal anastomotic vein.
5. Once the tube is placed in the correct position, the tube can be gently rotated until the conjunctiva is punctured and the orbital venous plexus is penetrated.
6. The tube is filled by capillary action.
7. Slight pressure may be placed over the eye to aid in hemostasis after the bleeding.
8. 0.5 ml may be collected from an adult mouse or gerbil.

Table 5-10
Hamster Complete Blood Count Reference Ranges

Erythrocytes	$5.0–10 \times 10^6/\mu l$
Hematocrit	36–55%
Hemoglobin	10–16 g/dl
Leukocytes	$6.3–8.9 \times 10^3/\mu l$
Neutrophils	10–42%
Lymphocytes	50–95%
Eosinophils	0–4.5%
Monocytes	0–3%
Basophils	0–1%
Platelets	$200–500 \times 10^6/\mu l$
Serum protein	5.9–6.5 g/dl
Albumin	2.63–4.10 g/dl
Globulin	2.7–4.2 g/dl

Table 5-11
Hamster Serum Biochemistry Reference Ranges

Serum glucose	60–150 mg/dl
Blood urea nitrogen	10–25 mg/dl
Creatinine	0.91–0.99 mg/dl
Total bilirubin	0.25–0.60 mg/dl
Cholesterol	25–135 mg/dl
Serum calcium	5–12 mg/dl
Serum phosphorus	3.4–8.2 mg/dl
Alkaline phosphatase	3.2–30.5 U/L
Alanine aminotransferase (ALT)	11.6–35.9 U/L
Aspartate aminotransferase (AST)	37.6–168 U/L

and *Spironucleus muris*.[3] *Hymenolepis diminuta* is a tapeworm that can cause constipation in hamsters.[3] This tapeworm can be detected during a fecal examination, at which time the owner must be informed that it is a zoonotic parasite.

Rodent pinworms, specifically *Syphacia muris* and *Syphacia obvelata,* are commonly diagnosed using the sticky side of clear cellophane tape to make an impression of the anus. The sticky surface will pick up the banana-shaped pinworm eggs, which can then be observed under a microscope.

PARASITOLOGY

Ectoparasites

Three species of mites are found in hamsters: *Demodex criceti, Demodex aurati*, and *Notoedres* spp.[6] *Notoedres* spp. is found around the hairless areas of the body: nose, ears, feet, and genitals.[6] *Spleorodens clethrionomys*, the nasal mite, and *Ornithonyssus bacoti*, the tropical rat mite, can also infest hamsters.[6] Diagnosis of ectoparasites in small rodents is similar to other species listed in this text. A skin scraping of the affected area will usually yield the parasite that needs to be treated.

Ivermectin is the drug of choice for ectoparasites in small mammals and pocket pets. Topical spot applications of amitraz, using a cotton-tipped applicator, work the best on very small mammals diagnosed with *Demodex* spp.

Internal Parasites

Hymenolepis nana, the dwarf tapeworm, can cause constipation in hamsters. Diagnosis can be made by finding individual eggs with polar bodies during fecal examination, or by finding the whole worm within the lumen of the small intestine during necropsy.[6]

As mentioned earlier, this is a zoonotic parasite and proper precautions should be taken regarding hygiene to prevent exposure after handling the animal. Recommended treatment for *H. nana* is praziquantel (Droncit, Haver/Diamond, Shawnee, KS, 5–10 mg/kg IM or SC).

THERAPEUTICS

(See guinea pig section.)

SURGICAL AND ANESTHETIC ASSISTANCE

(See guinea pig section.)

DISEASES

This section will review the common hamster diseases seen in veterinary practice. An overview of etiology, treatment, and prevention will follow a brief description of the disease presentation.

"WET-TAIL"

Diarrhea and gastrointestinal disorders in hamsters have been given a common name by the medical community and general public: wet-tail. There are a number of conditions and bacterial organisms that can contribute to this condition; but the primary organisms implicated in this disorder are different for young and adult animals.

In young hamsters (3–10 weeks old) proliferative ileitis is commonly caused by *Lawsonia intracellularis*.[7] This disease must be treated aggressively with fluid therapy, antibiotics, and force feeding. One of the recommended antibiotic regimes is enrofloxacin (10 mg/kg PO q12h for 5–7 days).[7] Fluid therapy is very important to combat electrolyte imbalances caused by diarrhea, dehydration, and anorexia. An electrolyte and glucose injection, at a dose of 40–60ml/kg SC q24h, should help maintain fluid and electrolyte levels within the body.[7] Force feeding a finely ground mixture of 1/2 fruits and vegetables and 1/2 hamster pellets, at a dose of 20–30 ml/kg q24h PO, will increase the caloric intake and energy level of the patient.[7]

When an improper antibiotic is selected to treat adult hamsters that present with diarrhea, normal flora can be killed, resulting in an overgrowth of *Clostridium difficile*. Penicillin, lincomycin, and bacitracin are all antibiotic choices that will contribute to the death of normal gut flora in hamsters, leading to enterotoxemia.[7]

Tyzzer's disease, caused by the bacterium *Clostridium piliforme*, brings about significant gastrointestinal illness in hamsters and gerbils, but not in rats and mice.[7] Tyzzer's disease is commonly transmitted between animals in displays and holding areas. This gastrointestinal bacterial infection primarily affects immunosuppressed, stressed animals.

NEOPLASIA

The average life span of a hamster is two years. The short life span and aging process increase the prevalence of tumors in these small rodents. If an animal is over 18 months of age, neoplastic disease should be considered as a differential diagnosis, especially if an asymmetrical mass is present. Treatment is removal of the affected tissue, if possible, to increase the quality of life for the small rodent.

OCULAR SYSTEM

Hamsters may present with one or both eyes protruding from the socket(s). If the animal is grabbed too tightly on the back of the neck, the eyes will start to bulge out of the sockets. If the eyes do prolapse from the socket, the eye and ocular area should be moistened with ophthalmic wash and lubricant (the lid margins retracted) and the globe gently returned to its normal anatomical location. The animal should then be maintained on antibiotic ophthalmic treatment for a week to 10 days.[7] If the problem reoccurs, a tarsorrhaphy or enucleation may be indicated.

GERBILS

One of the friendliest small rodent pets is the Mongolian gerbil (*Meriones unguiculatus*) (Figure 5-8). The most common color of pet gerbils is a tannish-brown (agouti), but other hair coat colors are available. If multiple animals are in the same enclosure with different hair coat colors, like-colored individuals will usually associate with each other.[1]

These animals are native to a very dry environment; therefore, they do not drink much water and produce little waste that would soil their environment. Regular cleaning of the enclosure is still encouraged to maintain healthy animals in an artificial setting. Food, water, and husbandry management is similar to other small rodents. (See the baseline gerbil physical information listed in Table 5-12.[2])

There is an androgen-dependent midventral scent gland on a gerbil's body. (See Table 5-12).[2] This scent gland should not be mistaken for an abnormal dermatologic lesion. A gerbil should be restrained by cupping a hand over the animal's back and immobilizing its head between the forefinger and middle finger, with the thumb supporting the rear of the animal. **Never attempt to restrain a gerbil by its tail, as the skin is easily removed (Figures 5-9A and 5-9B).**

DIAGNOSTIC SAMPLING

The collection of samples for diagnostic testing in gerbils is similar to the techniques used in other rodents. The reference ranges for complete blood counts and serum chemistry panels are listed in Tables 5-13 and 5-14.[2,3]

PARASITOLOGY

Gerbils are generally healthy animals; consequently, they are not very susceptible to parasite infestations. If parasites are suspected, follow the instructions for diagnostic testing used in other small rodents. *Demodex* spp. causing clinical dermatological lesions, including alopecia, has been reported.[4] Parasites are not a problem in healthy animals and underlying causes of immunosuppression must be investigated if they are diagnosed.

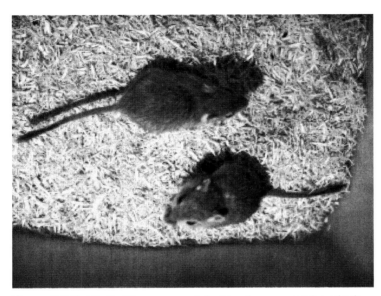

Figure 5-8 Gerbils. Gerbils are commonly kept together as companion animals.

DISEASES

"SORE NOSE"

Sore nose in gerbils is a disease condition thought to be caused by an increased secretion of porphyrins.[5] The harderian gland secretes porphyrins, which act as a primary skin irritant around the nasal opening. The irritated skin area is susceptible to secondary bacterial infections caused by *Staphylococcus* spp. Treating the resulting infectious dermatitis, and reducing stress to the animal, will usually resolve the problem.

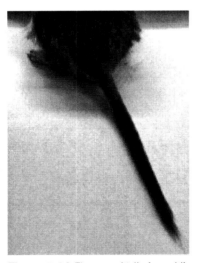

Figure 5-9A The normal tail of a gerbil.

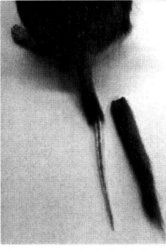

Figure 5-9B Tail skin slough. The skin can easily be removed if pulled when a gerbil is being captured.

Table 5-12
Gerbil Basic Information[1]

Body weight	Adult male	65–100 g
	Adult female	55–85 g
	Birth weight	2.5–3.5 g
Temperature, pulse and respiration	Rectal body temperature	99–101°F
	Normal heart rate	360 beats/minute
	Normal respiratory rate	90 breaths/minute
Amounts of food and water	Daily food consumption	5–8 g
	Daily water consumption	4 mL
Age at breeding initiation	Breeding initiation males	70–85 days
	Breeding initiation females	65–85 days
Female reproductive cycle	Estrous cycle	4 days (polyestrous)
	Gestation length (nonlactating)	24–26 days
	Gestation length (concurrent lactation)	27–48 days
	Litter size	3–7 (average 5) pups

EPILEPTIFORM SEIZURES

At around two months of age, 20–40% of gerbils develop epileptiform seizures.[5] There is no treatment for the seizures, which usually last for a few minutes, but do not appear to leave any permanent physical damage. As the animal ages, the seizure activity declines in severity and occurrence.

Table 5-13
Gerbil Complete Blood Count Reference Ranges

Erythrocytes	$7.0–10 \times 10^6/\mu l$
Hematocrit	41–52%
Hemoglobin	12.1–16.9 g/dl
Leukocytes	$4.3–21.6 \times 10^3/\mu l$
Neutrophils	5–34%
Lymphocytes	60–95%
Eosinophils	0–4%
Monocytes	0–3%
Basophils	0–1%
Platelets	$400–600 \times 10^6/\mu l$
Serum protein	4.3–12.5 g/dl
Albumin	1.8–5.5 g/dl
Globulin	1.6–6.0 g/dl

Table 5-14
Gerbil Serum Biochemistry Reference Ranges

Serum glucose	50–135 mg/dl
Blood urea nitrogen	17–27 mg/dl
Creatinine	0.6–1.47 mg/dl
Total bilirubin	0.2–0.6 mg/dl
Cholesterol	90–150 mg/dl
Serum calcium	3.7–6.2 mg/dl
Serum phosphorus	3.7–7.0 mg/dl

RATS

Rats, like mice, are common laboratory animals and are also propagated for reptile food. Unlike mice, rats have excellent pet characteristics that include a personable disposition and a charming intelligence. The common rat species maintained as a companion animal is *Rattus norvegicus,* with the white rat and hooded rat being the most common variations (Figure 5-10). Although rats have an excellent temperament for companionship, they can inflict a serious bite if provoked. Also, as with other animal species, humans can be allergic to their hair, skin dander, urine, and salivary proteins.[2] Rats are not as territorial as other rodent species and are very social. Food, water, and husbandry management is similar to that of other small rodents. (Refer to the baseline rat physical information listed in Table 5-15.[1,2])

Rats are continuous, polyestrous rodents that should be bred in polygamous or monogamous set-ups, due to the males' aggressive territoriality behavior.[1] When breeding rats in a polygamous ratio, there may be one male with 2–6 females. Females are removed from a polygamous cage prior to parturition. A monogamous pair is maintained together with the young until weaning.

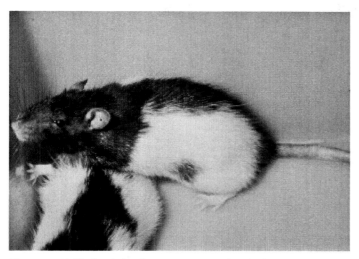

To restrain a rat, the animal should be picked up with one hand placed over the animal's back and rib cage, while restraining its head with the thumb and forefinger directly behind its jaws. The other hand grasps the tail, stabilizing the animal. As with other rodents, the skin on the dorsal cervical region may also be used to pick up a rat.

Figure 5-10 The hooded rat is a common type of rat that is kept as a pet.

Table 5-15
Rat Basic Information[1,2]

Body weight	Adult male	450–520 grams
	Adult female	250–320 grams
	Birth weight	5–6 grams
Temperature, pulse and respiration	Rectal body temperature	99–101°F
	Normal heart rate	250–450 beats/minute
	Normal respiratory rate	70–115 breaths/minute
Amounts of food and water	Daily food consumption	10 grams/100 grams body weight
	Daily water consumption	10–12 ml/100 grams body weight
Age at onset of puberty and breeding life	Sexual maturity, male	65–110 days
	Sexual maturity, female	65–110 days
Female reproductive cycle	Estrous cycle	4–5 days
	Gestation length	21–23 days
	Litter size	6–12

DIAGNOSTIC SAMPLING

The collection of samples for diagnostic testing in rats is similar to the techniques used in other rodents. The reference ranges for complete blood counts and serum chemistry panels are listed in Tables 5-16 and 5-17.[2,3]

PARASITOLOGY

Specific parasites identified in rats include the dwarf tapeworm (*Hymenolepis nana*), pinworms (*Syphacia muris*), nematodes (specifically, *Trichosomoides crassicauda*), *Giardia muris*, and the following ectoparasites: *Ornithonyssus bacotic* (the tropical rat mite), *Radfordia ensifera* (the rat fur mite), *Demodex nanus*, *Polyplax spinulosa* (the spined rat louse), and fleas. Diagnosis and treatments are similar to those recommended for mice, although the dosages and duration will differ.

Diseases

BACTERIAL AND VIRAL INFECTIONS

Staphylococcus aureus is the most common cause of ulcerative dermatitis in rats.[7] *Mycoplasma pulmonis*, *Streptococcus pneumoniae*, *Corynebacterium kutscheri*, Sendai virus and cilia-associated respiratory bacillus have been isolated and identified as infectious agents causing rat respiratory disease. With respiratory pathogens, clinical signs can vary from mild dyspnea to severe pneumonia and death. The treatment of mycoplasmosis in rats is similar to that of infected mice.

TUMORS

Rats are very susceptible to tumors, most likely due to the animals' short life span and physiologic predisposition. The most common subcutaneous tumor in rats is the fibroadenoma of the mammary tissue.[7] Mammary tumors can reach very large sizes and affect both males and females. To reduce the incidence of fibroadenomas, overiohysterectomies are advocated at an early age in female rats. Whereas mammary tumors in mice are almost always malignant, rat mammary tumors are usually localized and respond to surgical resection.

Table 5-16
Rat Complete Blood Count Reference Ranges

Erythrocytes	$5.4–8.5 \times 10^6/mm^3$
Hematocrit	37–49%
Hemoglobin	11.5–16 mg/dl
Leukocytes	$6.6–12.6 \times 10^3/mm^3$
Neutrophils	$1.77–3.38 \times 10^3/mm^3$
Lymphocytes	$4.78–9.12 \times 10^3/mm^3$
Eosinophils	$0.03–0.08 \times 10^3/mm^3$
Monocytes	$0.01–0.04 \times 10^3/mm^3$
Basophils	$0.00–0.03 \times 10^3/mm^3$
Platelets	$150–460 \times 10^6/mm^3$
Serum protein	5.6–7.6 g/dl
Albumin	3.8–4.8 g/dl
Globulin	1.8–3.0 g/dl

Table 5-17
Rat Serum Biochemistry Reference Ranges

Serum glucose	50–135 mg/dl
Blood urea nitrogen	15–21 mg/dl
Creatinine	0.2–0.8 mg/dl
Total bilirubin	0.20–0.55 mg/dl
Cholesterol	40–130 mg/dl
Serum calcium	7.2–13.9 mg/dl
Serum phosphate	3.11–11.0 mg/dl
Alkaline phosphatase	56.8–128 U/L
Alanine aminotransferase (ALT)	17.5–30.2 U/L
Aspartate aminotransferase (AST)	45.7–80.8 U/L

SIALODACRYOADENITIS VIRUS

This virus is a cornavirus that affects the cervical salivary glands and sometimes the lacrimal glands of the eye. The cervical lymph nodes can become enlarged and the eyes may protrude if the lacrimal gland(s) is affected. There is no treatment for this highly contagious disease.

MICE

Although not a common companion animal, mice (*Mus musculus*) are maintained in captive conditions as pets and for reptile food. The African pygmy mouse is another genus of mouse that is commonly maintained as a pet.[2] There are a number of behavioral and physical characteristics that make mice undesirable pets. These include: aggressive, protective behavior often resulting in painful bites to the owner; territorial behavior that often results in severe injury to cage mates; potential human allergies to the hair and skin dander; and a strong, undesirable smell to the urine. Even with these undesirable characteristics, mice can be good pets for owners who are willing to work with the animals and accept their negative aspects (Figure 5-11).

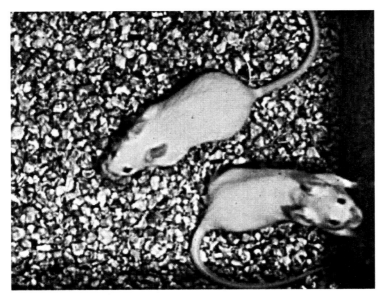

Mice are maintained in environments that are similar to other small rodents, but a thorough cage cleaning is required more often—because of their smelly urine. Food, water, and husbandry management is similar to that of other small rodents listed in this chapter.

Figure 5-11 Mice in cage. Mice are sometimes maintained as companion animals.

Mice are continuous, polyestrous rodents that should be bred in polygamous or monogamous set-ups, due to the males' aggressive, territorial behavior (Figure 5-12).[1] When breeding mice in a polygamous ratio, there may be one male with 2–6 females. Females are removed from a polygamous cage prior to parturition. A monogamous pair is maintained together with the young until weaning.

To restrain a mouse, the tail should be grabbed with the thumb and forefinger, allowing the mouse to hold on to an object with its front feet. When the mouse securely attaches itself to an object, the other hand then grabs the skin at the dorsal skin in the cervical region, while keeping the tail in a firm grasp.

DIAGNOSTIC SAMPLING

The collection of samples for diagnostic testing in mice is similar to techniques used in other rodents. The reference ranges for complete blood counts and serum chemistry panels are listed in Tables 5-18 and 5-19.[1,2]

PARASITOLOGY

There are a number of parasites that have been identified in mice. *Hymenolepis nana* (the dwarf tapeworm) and *Cysticercus fasciolaris* (the larval stage of the cat tapeworm) can be isolated from these small rodents. The dwarf tapeworm is often found in young mice that are dead or in mice that present with severe gastroenteritis (resulting in diarrhea). Diagnosis of the dwarf tapeworm can be made with a fecal flotation exam or by finding the tapeworms in the small intestine at necropsy. Dwarf tapeworm can be treated with praziquantal.

Syphacia oblevata are commensal oxyurid nematodes that feed on bacteria that inhabit the intestinal tract of mice.[6] Although nonpathogenic in most cases, an overwhelming number can cause severe irritation of the terminal gastrointestinal tract. These nematode parasites can be diagnosed using transparent tape and applying it to the rectal area. After removing the tape from the affected rectal area, it can be placed on a slide and the ova viewed under a microscope. Ivermectin and fenbendazole have been used effectively in treating this parasite in mice.[6]

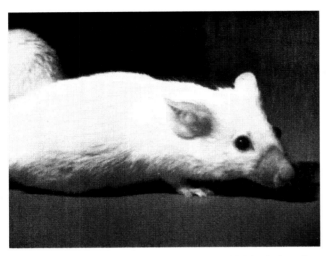

Figure 5-12 Mice are very territorial and may exhibit barbering when kept together. Barbering is defined as the physiological removal of hair by a cagemate through biting.

Giardia muris is a common protozoal parasite that affects mice. This organism can be seen using a direct fecal examination. Metronidazole is the treatment of choice for *Giardia* infections in small rodents.

Ectoparasitism in mice is a presentation that clinicians often see and diagnose. *Myobia musculi, Myocoptes musculinis, Radfordia affinis,* and *Psoregates simplex* are

Table 5-18
Mouse Basic Information[1,2]

Body weight	Adult male	20–40 grams
	Adult female	25–40 grams
	Birth weight	0.8–2.0 grams
Temperature, pulse and respiration	Rectal body temperature	97–100°F
	Normal heart rate	325–780 beats/minute
	Normal respiratory rate	60–220 breaths/minute
Amounts of food and water	Daily food consumption	15 g/100 g body weight
	Daily water consumption	15 ml/100 g body weight
Age at onset of puberty and breeding life	Sexual maturity, male	50 days
	Sexual maturity, female	50–60 days
Female reproductive cycle	Estrous cycle	4–5 days
	Gestation length	19–21 days
	Litter size	10–12

Table 5-19
Mouse Complete Blood Count Reference Ranges

Erythrocytes	$7.0–12.5 \times 10^6/mm^3$
Hematocrit	36–49%
Hemoglobin	10.2–18 mg/dl
Leukocytes	$6–15 \times 10^3/mm^3$
Neutrophils	10–40%
Lymphocytes	55–95%
Eosinophils	0–4%
Monocytes	0.1–3.5%
Basophils	0–0.3%
Platelets	$160–410 \times 10^6/mm^3$
Serum protein	3.5–7.2 g/dl
Albumin	2.5–4.8 g/dl
Globulin	1.8–3.0 g/dl

all mice fur mites that can cause severe self-mutilation and hair loss. *Polyplax serrata*, the house mouse louse, can cause anemia, pruritus, dermatitis, and death.[6] Diagnosis of ectoparasites in mice is similar to that used in other companion animal species. Treatment of ectoparasites can be accomplished with ivermectin and topical mitacide. As with other rodent species, there appears to be an increasing resistance to ivermectin by ectoparasites.

Diseases

BARBERING

Barbering is a condition in which a cagemate bites fur from the affected area to the skin without causing any dermatological damage. This condition is usually caused by stress induced from overcrowding or due to the establishment of a hierarchy within the group.

TUMORS

As with many small rodents, mammary tumors are a common presentation in older female mice. The most common mammary tumor found in mice is the adenocarcinoma.[7]

BACTERIAL AND VIRAL INFECTIONS

Bacterial infections associated with dermatitis lesions and subcutaneous abscesses in mice are commonly caused by *Staphylococcus aureus*, *Pasteurella pneumontropica,* and *Streptococcus pyogens*.[7] Acute and chronic respiratory infections may be caused by Sendai virus or *Mycoplasma pulmonis*, but are most commonly associated with Sendai virus, from which adults survive but neonates often die. Chronic respiratory infections—with clinical signs of pneumonia, suppurative rhinitis, and occasionally, otitis media—may be the result of a *Mycoplasma pulmonis* infection. Both infections should be treated using supportive care, while mycoplasmosis can be treated specifically with enrofloxacin in combination with doxycycline hyclate for 7 days.[7]

REFERENCES

Guinea Pig References

1. Harkness, J.E. *Pet Rodents: A Guide for Practitioners.* AAHA Press, 1997.
2. Johnson-Delaney, C.A. and Harrison, L.R. *Guinea Pigs. Exotic Companion Medicine Handbook for Veterinarians.* Lake Worth, Florida: Wingers Publishing, 1996: 1–20.
3. Hillyer, E.V., Quesenberry, K.E., and Donnelly , T.M. "Guinea Pigs and Chinchillas, Biology, Husbandry and Clinical Techniques." In Hillyer, E.V. and Quesenberry, K.E. eds., *Ferrets, Rabbits and Rodents: Clinical Medicine and Surgery.* Philadelphia: W.B. Saunders, 1997: 243–59.
4. Cualiffe-Beamer, T. and Les, E. "The Laboratory Mouse." In Poole, T.B. ed., *The UFAW Handbook on the Care and Management of Laboratory Animals.* Essex: Longman Scientific & Technical, 1994: 290–1.
5. Chrisp, C.E., Suckow, M.A., Fayer, R. et al., "Comparison of the Host Ranges and Antigenicity of *Cryptosporidium parvum* and *Cryptosporidium wrairi* from Guinea Pigs," *J Protozool*, 39 (1992) 406–9.
6. Schaeffer, D.O. and Donnelly, T.M. "Disease Problems of Guinea Pigs and Chinchillas." In Hillyer, E.V. and Quesenberry, K.E. eds., *Ferrets, Rabbits and Rodents: Clinical Medicine*

and Surgery. Philadelphia: W.B. Saunders, 1997: 260–81.

7. Adamcak, A. and Otten, B. "Rodent Therapeutics," *Vet Clinics of North America. Exotic Animal Practice*, 3 (January 2000) 221–35.

8. Mullen, H. "Soft tissue Surgery." In Hillyer, E.V. and Quesenberry, K.E. eds., *Ferrets, Rabbits and Rodents: Clinical Medicine and Surgery*, Philadelphia: W.B. Saunders, 1997: 283–8.

9. Mason, D.E. "Anesthesia, Analgesia and Sedation for Small Mammals." In Hillyer, E.V. and Quesenberry, K.E. eds., *Ferrets, Rabbits and Rodents: Clinical Medicine and Surgery.* Philadelphia: W.B. Saunders, 1997: 378–91.

Hamster, Rat, and Mouse References

1. Johnson-Delaney, C.A. and Harrison, L.R. *Small Rodent: Exotic Companion Medicine Handbook for Veterinarians.* Lake Worth, Florida: Winger's Publishing, 1996: 48–61.

2. Harkness, J.E. *Pet Rodents: A Guide for Practitioners.* AAHA Press, 1997: 27–30.

3. McClure, D.E. "Clinical Pathology and Sample Collection in the Laboratory Rodent." *Vet Clinics of North America. Exotic Animal Practice*, 2 (September 1999): 565–90.

4. Silverman, J. "Biomethodology." In Vantloosier, G.L., Jr. and McPherson, E.W. eds., *Laboratory Hamsters.* Orlando, Florida: Academic Press, 1987: 70–94.

5. Bauck, L. and Bihun, C. "Small Rodents, Basic Anatomy, Physiology, Husbandry, and Clinical Techniques." In Hillyer, E.V. and Quesenberry, K.E. eds., *Ferrets, Rabbits and Rodents: Clinical Medicine and Surgery.* Philadelphia: W.B. Saunders, 1997: 291–306.

6. Morrisey, J.K. "Parasites of Ferrets, Rabbits and Rodents," Seminar on Avian Exotic Pet Medicine, 5 (1996) 106–14.

7. Donelly, T.M. "Disease Problems of Small Rodents." In Hillyer, E.V. and Quesenberry K.E. eds., *Ferrets, Rabbits and Rodents: Clinical Medicine and Surgery.* Philadelphia: W.B. Saunders, 1997: 307–25.

Gerbil References

1. Wong, R., Gray-Allan, P., Chifa, C., and Alfred, B. "Social Preference of Female Gerbils (*Meriones unguiculatus*) As Influenced by Coat Color of Males," *Behavioral Neural Biology*, 54 (1990): 184–190.

2. Johnson-Delaney, C.A. and Harrison, L.R. *Small Rodents: Exotic Companion Medicine Handbook for Veterinarians.* Lake Worth, Florida: Wingers Publishing, 1996: 38–46.

3. Bauck, L. and Bihun, C. "Small Rodents, Basic Anatomy, Physiology, Husbandry and Clinical Techniques." In Hillyer, E.V. and Quesenberry, K.E. eds., *Ferrets, Rabbits and Rodents: Clinical Medicine and Surgery.* Philadelphia: W.B. Saunders, 1997: 291–306.

4. Morrisey, J.K. "Parasites of Ferrets, Rabbits and Rodents," Seminar on Avian Exotic Pet Medicine 5, (2) (1996) 106–14.

5. Donnelly, T.M. "Disease Problems of Small Rodents." In Hillyer, E.V. and Quesenberry, K.E. eds., *Ferrets, Rabbits and Rodents: Clinical Medicine and Surgery.* Philadelphia: W.B. Saunders, 1997: 307–25

CHAPTER 6

HEDGEHOGS

INTRODUCTION

Hedgehogs are mammals that are covered with spines over their entire bodies except their faces and bellies (Figures 6-1A and 6-1B). These animals have gained in popularity as small companion animals over the last 5–10 years, despite their spiny anatomy. The most common pet species is the white-bellied, four-toed African or African pygmy hedgehog (*Atelerix albiventris*).[1] Unfortunately, most pet hedgehogs are nocturnal, shy, and prefer quiet environments. If startled or frightened, the animal will either "ball-up" with its back spines elevated or will try to hide. As these animals age, they will learn to accept an owner, but will rarely develop the trust displayed by other small mammals. As with other animals, it

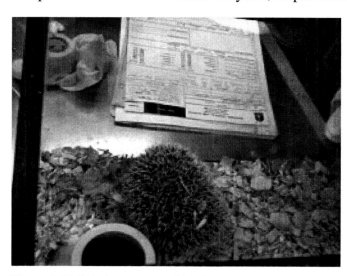

Figure 6-1A Hedgehogs are covered in spines.

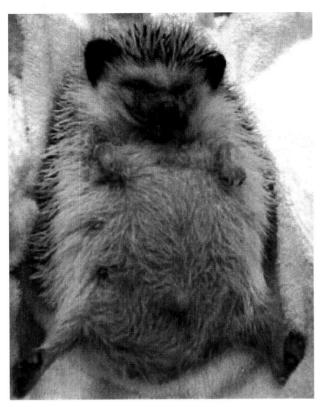

Figure 6-1B Hedgehogs, however, do not have spines on their faces or abdomens.

is important for the technician to know the normal physiologic values in order to assess the patient's health status (Table 6-1).

A hedgehog, when presented with a new object, may perform a ritual called self-anointing. The animal first licks the object, then begins to hypersalivate. This frothy saliva is then rubbed on its skin and spines; the purpose of this ritual is unknown.[3]

Hedgehogs are territorial, as are most small mammals; therefore, close monitoring for fighting is required when a new animal is introduced to a group within an enclosure.

Table 6-1
Hedgehog Basic Information[2]

Average life span		3–5 years
Body weight	Adult male	500–600 grams
	Adult female	250–400 grams
	Birth weight	average 10 grams
Temperature	Rectal body temperature	97–98°F
Female reproductive info.	Gestation length	34–37 days
	Litter size	3 average

HUSBANDRY

ENVIRONMENTAL CONCERNS

Pet hedgehogs can be maintained in the environmental temperatures favored by human inhabitants of the house. Extremely cold or hot environmental temperatures will cause these animals stress and a depressed psychological state. The preferred housing for these small, spiny animals is a glass-sided enclosure with a commercial screen top that can be secured with tabs or screws. The "hedgehog house" should have enough floor surface area to include a small hiding box, a specific hedgehog exercise wheel (wire wheels are dangerous), and a pan or shallow dish for swimming. The cage substrate of choice is shredded newspaper or a pelleted paper product. Wood chips, ground corncob, ground walnut shell, and cloth towels are not recommended for hedgehog cage flooring.

NUTRITION

Hedgehogs need fresh water daily. Although they can learn to drink from sipper tubes, a small shallow dish may be preferred as a water container. These animals are naturally insectivores/omnivores and their diet should reflect their dietary wants and nutritional needs. There may be a commercial pelleted hedgehog diet available and this should be used with supplements of vegetables, fruits, and insects. A recommended diet for adult hedgehogs is listed below in Table 6-2, and should be followed if a commercial diet is not available.

Table 6-2
Hedgehog Daily Diet[2]

1. 3 heaping teaspoons high-quality cat/kitten chow
2. 1 heaping teaspoon fruit/vegetable mix
Finely chop all ingredients and mix together:
½ teaspoon leafy dark greens (spinach, kale, leaf lettuce),
¼ teaspoon diced carrot, ¼ teaspoon diced apple,
¼ teaspoon diced banana, ¼ teaspoon diced grape or raisin,
and ¼ teaspoon vitamin/mineral powder (e.g., Vionate[®])
3. 6 small mealworms or 1-2 crickets

RESTRAINT

The spines on these small mammals make restraint difficult. It is recommended to wear lightweight leather gloves to prevent injury to the technician or veterinarian examining the patient. Some hedgehogs are docile enough to be examined without "balling up," but there is always a possibility that they will become frightened and curl, causing pain to the handler. Most hedgehog patients need to be anesthetized with isoflurane anesthesia for the physical examination process. General anesthesia is quick and, in most cases, reduces stress to the animal and handler. The patient is induced in an induction chamber and then maintained using a small mask. Since hedgehogs ball up when frightened, it is almost impossible to mask these animals without first inducing in a chamber or using an injectable preanesthetic medication (Table 6-3).

Table 6-3
Injectable Anesthetic Agents Used in Hedgehogs[4]

Drug	Route	Dosage
Ketamine	IM	5–20 mg/kg
Ketamine and Diazepam	IM	5–20 mg/kg (Ketamine) 0.5–2 mg/kg (Diazepam)
Ketamine and Xylazine	IM	10–20 mg/kg (Ketamine) 2 mg/kg (Xylazine)

Other methods have been used to uncurl and examine these animals without using general anesthesia. These physical handling techniques are not recommended unless the animal is very ill or docile.

PHYSICAL EXAMINATION

The animal must be properly restrained. It is important that the technician and/or veterinarian be able to examine the entire animal without a concern for being stuck by quills. A complete physical examination should be performed on each hedgehog patient that enters the clinic. The questions used to obtain the clinical history and physical examination procedures for hedgehogs are similar to those used for other small mammals.

DIAGNOSTIC SAMPLING

BLOOD COLLECTION

Using a 3-cc syringe with a 1/4" 26-gauge needle, blood samples may be collected from the superficial veins, including the lateral saphenous and cephalic vein. For larger volumes of blood, the jugular vein, cranial vena cava, and femoral veins may be used. Blood for diagnostic sampling is easier to obtain from an anesthetized hedgehog than one that is being manually restrained. Reference ranges for complete blood counts and serum chemistry panels are listed in Tables 6-4 and 6-5.[5]

Table 6-4
Hedgehog Complete Blood Count Reference Ranges

Erythrocytes	$4.4–6.0 \times 10^6/\mu L$
Hematocrit	28–38%
Hemoglobin	9.9–13.1 g/dL
Leukocytes	$5.8–21.0 \times 10^3/\mu L$
Neutrophils	49–70%
Lymphocytes	22–38%
Eosinophils	2–11%
Monocytes	0%
Basophils	0–5%
Platelets	$200–412 \times 10^3/\mu L$
Serum protein	5.3–6.3 g/dL
Albumin	3.4–3.6 g/dL

Table 6-5
Hedgehog Serum Biochemistry Reference Ranges

Serum glucose	81.5–116.1 mg/dl
Blood urea nitrogen	21.3–32.9 mg/dl
Creatinine	0.2–0.4 mg/dl
Total bilirubin	0–0.1 mg/dl
Serum calcium	9.5–10.9 mg/dl
Serum phosphorus	4.7–6.5 mg/dl
Alanine aminotransferase (ALT)	39.7–68.9 IU/L

OTHER DIAGNOSTIC TECHNIQUES

Although no normal urinalysis values have been published for hedgehogs, urine may be collected by cystocentesis, catheterization, or free catch.[4] Abnormal findings in hedgehog urine include white blood cells, neoplastic cells, and cystralluria.[4]

Other diagnostic procedures that need to be performed on hedgehogs are done in a manner similar to those used with other small mammals.

PARASITOLOGY

Ectoparasites

A common clinical presentation is quill loss due to *Caparinia tripilis*, the common mange mite of hedgehogs.[6] Pruritus, quill loss, and hyperkeratosis are commonly associated with a quill mite infestation. Diagnosis can be made through skin scrapings of the affected area. As with most small mammals, ivermectin treatment alone is not effective in treating mite infestations. Amitraz (0.3% topically once every seven days for 2 or 3 treatments) in conjunction with ivermectin (0.2–0.4 mg/kg orally or subcutaneously every 10–14 days for 2 or 3 treatments) is the recommended treatment for mites. For an effective treatment, owners must clean the environment at least every two days to prevent reinfestation.

Other mite species, including *Chorioptes* spp., fleas, and ticks are also external parasites that may be found on hedgehogs.[5] Treatment and prevention are similar to those used with other small mammals.

Internal Parasites

Routine fecal floatation and direct fecal parasite examinations are used to diagnose internal parasites. *Isospora eriniacei* and *Eimeria rastegaiv* are the common coccidian parasites identified in hedgehogs.[4] To treat coccidia, sulfadimethoxine is recommended (2 to 20 mg/kg, per os daily for 2 to 5 days, skip 5 days and repeat).[4]

Commonly identified nematode species include the lungworm (*Crenosoma striatum*), intestinal nematodes (*Capillaria erinacei*), tapeworms (*Hymenolepis erinacei*), and flukes (*Brachylaemus erinacei*). Treatment of choice for nematodes is fenbendazole (10–25 mg/

kg per os) or ivermectin (0.2 mg/kg subcutaneously or per os).[4] Cestodes should be treated with praziquantel (7 mg/kg subcutaneously or per os).[4]

THERAPEUTICS

Since hedgehogs are covered with spines and go into a defensive posture when upset, treatment can be difficult. Oral medications that are flavored to be palatable are the recommended treatments of choice. The patient thus readily accepts the treatment without stress and trauma. If subcutaneous injections are being used, tissue absorption can be affected by the thick fat layer under the skin.

Since hedgehog veins are short and small, an intraosseous catheter placed in the femur is recommended for critical patients. The approach is through the trochanteric fossa with a 20- or 22-gauge 1.5" spinal needle.[7]

DISEASES

This section will review the common hedgehog diseases seen in veterinary practice. An overview of etiology, treatment, and prevention will follow a brief description of the disease presentation.

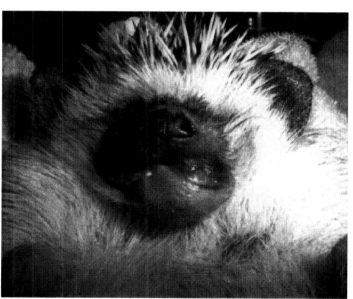

Figure 6-2 Oral mass. Tumors are often seen in pet hedgehogs.

NEOPLASIA

One of the most common disease presentations affecting hedgehogs is neoplasia (Figure 6-2). There is not a specific neoplastic disease that affects hedgehogs; therefore, any abnormal mass should be biopsied for disease determination. Some internal neoplasias can present as nonspecific disease presentations, so all sick hedgehogs must have a complete diagnostic work-up. As with other animal species, the older the animal, the more predisposed it is to neoplastic disease—which, in the case of hedgehogs, is over 3 years old.

DERMATOMYCOSES

Fungal organisms that are often identified as infecting hedgehogs are *T. mentagrophytes*, *T. erinacei,* and *Microsporum* spp.[5] These organisms can be diagnosed as a single infection or a concurrent infection with a mite infestation. Diagnosis is established by culturing spines from the affected areas in DTM media. Systemic treatment of oral griseofulvin is recommended at (30 to 40 mg/kg once daily for 30 days).[5]

RESPIRATORY DISEASE

Bordetella bronchiseptica, Pasteurella multocida, and *Coryenbacterium pneumonia* have been identified as respiratory pathogens affecting hedgehogs. Routine diagnostics to identify the causative agent of the respiratory disease is required for proper treatment. Treatment for severe respiratory disease includes antibiotics (based on culture and sensitivity of the causative agent), supportive fluid therapy, oxygen therapy, and nebulization.[4]

REFERENCES

1. Smith, A.J. "Husbandry and Nutrition of Hedgehogs." *Vet Clinics of North America (Exotic Animal Practice)* 2, no.1, 1999: 127–141.

2. Johnson-Delaney, C. and Harrison, L.R. *Hedgehogs: Exotic Companion Medicine Handbook for Veterinarians.* Lake Worth, Florida: Wingers Publishing, 1996: 1–14.

3. Hoefer, H.L. "Hedgehogs." *Vet Clinics of North America (Small Animal Practice)* 24, no.1 (1994): 113–120.

4. Larsen, R.S. and Carpenter, J.W. "Husbandry and Medical Management of African Hedgehogs." *Veterinary Medicine* (October 1999): 877–888.

5. Ness, R.D. "Clinical Pathology and Sample Collection of Exotic Small Mammals." *Vet Clinics of North America (Exotic Animal Practice)* 2, no. 3 (1999): 591–620.

6. Gerson, L. and Boever, W.J. "Acariasis (*Caparinia* spp.) in Hedgehogs (*Erinaceus* spp.): Diagnosis and Treatment." *Journal of Zoo Animal Medicine* 14 (1983): 17–19.

7. Brown, SA. and Rosenthal, K.L. *Self-Assessment Color Review of Small Mammals.* Ames, Iowa: Iowa State University Press, 1997: 14–15.

CHAPTER 7

SUGAR GLIDERS

INTRODUCTION

The sugar or honey glider (*Petaurus breviceps*) is a marsupial that is native to New Guinea and Australia (Figure 7-1). It is about the size of a North American flying squirrel, generally gray in color with a black stripe running along the dorsal surface from the nose to the base of the tail. These animals have some control of the tail, which can be used as a rudder during gliding or for carrying nest material up a tree. The second and third digits of each hind foot are partially fused forming a "hair comb," which is used for grooming their soft fur.

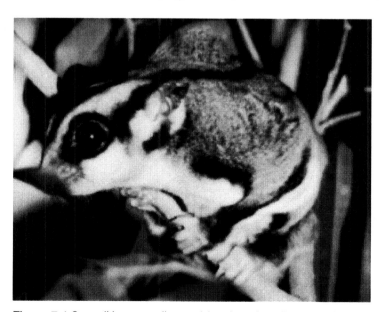

Figure 7-1 Sugar gliders are small marsupials native to Australia and New Guinea.

The male sugar gliders have three scent glands: one on top of the head (which forms a bald spot upon maturation), another on the chest (causing an orange or rusty discoloration of fur in that area), and one in the anal area. The testicles are located in a furry pouch in the midventral, and a bifurcated penis is ventral to the base of the tail.

The female has a pouch, or marsupium, located on the ventral aspect of the body where the young are raised (Figure 7-2). Female sugar gliders do not have the bald scent gland (on top of the head) that is found on males of this species.

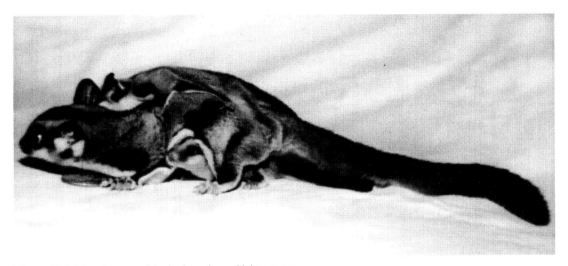

Figure 7-2 A female sugar glider is shown here with her young.

Sugar gliders can bark, making a yipping sound, or screech. Some have compared the screeching sound to that of an electric pencil sharpener. Sugar gliders are nocturnal animals, as evidenced by their extremely large eyes. Since these animals are awake at night, they have a tendency to bark—especially the males during a full moon. Leaving a light on in an adjacent room will help reduce this bothersome behavior early in the morning (3:00 A.M.). As with other animals, it is important for the technician to know the normal physiologic values in order to assess the patient's health status (Table 7-1).

Table 7-1
Sugar Glider Basic Information[1]

Body weight	Adult male	115–160 grams
	Adult female	95–135 grams
	Birth weight	0.19 grams
Temperature	Rectal body temperature	97.2°F
Female reproductive info.	Sexual maturity	8–15 months
	Gestation length	15–17 days
	Litter size	1–2 average
	Pouch emergence	60–70 days
	Weaning age	110–120 days
	Average life span (captive)	10 years

These animals are extremely sensitive to pesticides, cedar shavings, branches from toxic trees, and bright direct light (either artificial or sunlight). Dogs and cats should be kept at a distance, and strict supervision must be maintained when sugar gliders are handled by small children or released from their enclosure.

HUSBANDRY

Cage dimensions for sugar gliders should be at least 18" x 18" x 24" with the size of the wire openings not more than 0.5–1.0". Any cage material that meets the above dimensions will work, but, to prevent trauma, the owner must be sure no protruding wires or openings are found within the enclosure. A pine box approximately 6" x 8" x 6" is needed for the animal to sleep in during the day. This can be a premanufactured bird nesting box. Shredded paper makes an excellent nontoxic box substrate. Old towels or cloth can unravel, leaving loose strings to choke the animal or strangulate a foot or tail. Tree branches need to be included in the enclosure for the animal to climb on during its play and exercise time. The branches can be obtained from nontoxic species of hardwood trees.

NUTRITION

Two food dishes and a sipper bottle should be used to feed and provide water for sugar gliders. One food dish is used for dry food, while the other is for moist food (Figure 7-3).

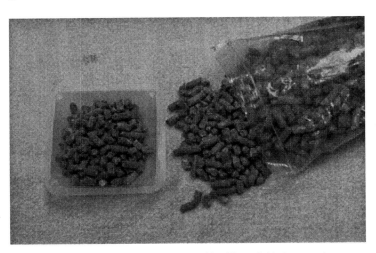

A balanced diet of 75% fruits and vegetables and 25% protein will often ensure good health for these animals. Sugar gliders should have low-fat diets, with no access to refined sugars, chocolate, or processed human foods with preservatives. Sunflower seed, corn, cat food (dry, light diet), a dog biscuit, and a salt/mineral block should be maintained in the cage at all times. Once

Figure 7-3 Sugar glider food. Manufactured food is available to prevent common health problems associated with malnutrition.

a month, a monkey biscuit soaked in apple juice should be placed in the cage for additional nutritional benefit. Vitamin supplements, such as Repti-Cal® and Herptivite®, should be sprinkled on fruits and vegetables every 3 to 4 days. Chicken, or chicken flavored dog food (with honey wheat germ sprinkled on top), Nekton Lori® (5 parts water to 1 part Nekton), and a hard-boiled egg with the shell (1/8 per animal) should also be offered.

Two or three of the following offerings should be fed each day.

1. grated carrot/apple/raisin salad

2. mixed frozen vegetables

3. fresh vegetables

4. natural applesauce

5. Beechnut® baby food – meat and/or vegetables

6. cooked pasta, unsalted crackers, toasted whole wheat bread

7. mealworms, crickets, waxworms

RESTRAINT

Sugar gliders are restrained by holding the head between the thumb and middle finger and resting the index finger on top of its head.[1] The body will then lie in the palm of the restrainer's hand. Isoflurane anesthesia is the agent of choice for general anesthesia of these small marsupials. Placing the patient in an induction chamber using 5% isoflurane with 1.5 L flow of oxygen will allow the animal to become anesthetized with minimal stress. The animal can then be maintained on approximately 2–3% isoflurane using a facemask and 1.5 L flow of oxygen.

PHYSICAL EXAMINATION

The animal must be properly restrained. It is important that the technician and/or veterinarian be able to examine the entire animal without stress to the patient or examiner. A complete physical examination should be performed on each sugar glider patient that enters the clinic. The questions used to obtain the clinical history and physical examination procedures for sugar gliders are similar to those used for other small mammals.

DIAGNOSTIC SAMPLING

BLOOD COLLECTION

Recommended sites for blood collection, which is best accomplished under general anesthesia, are the jugular vein, cranial vena cava, or medial tibial artery.[1] Blood volumes of up to 1% of the animal's body weight may be safely collected using a 3-cc syringe and a 26-gauge needle. Reference ranges for complete blood counts and serum chemistry panels are listed in Tables 7-2 and 7-3.[1]

Other diagnostic procedures performed on sugar gliders are done in a manner similar to those used with other small mammals.

PARASITOLOGY

Although common in wild sugar gliders, parasites are not commonly diagnosed in captive-bred animals. Coccidia and *Giardia* spp. have been identified in animals raised in captivity.[2]

Table 7-2
Sugar Glider Complete Blood Count Reference Ranges

Erythrocytes	7–$8.8 \times 10^6/\mu l$
Hematocrit	39.7–47.7%
Hemoglobin	13.9–17.1 g/dl
Leukocytes	2.1–$8.5 \times 10^3/\mu l$
Neutrophils	0.2–$2.4 \times 10^3/\mu l$
Lymphocytes	1.6–$6.0 \times 10^3/\mu l$
Eosinophils	0.04–$0.16 \times 10^3/\mu l$
Monocytes	0–$3 \times 10^3/\mu l$
Platelets	602–$904 \times 10^3/\mu l$
Serum protein	5.4–6.6 g/dl
Albumin	4.4–4.8 g/dl
Globulin	1.5–1.9 g/dl

Table 7-3
Sugar Glider Serum Biochemistry Reference Ranges

Serum glucose	76–232 mg/dl
Blood urea nitrogen	1–89 mg/dl
Creatinine	0.6–0.8 mg/dl
Total bilirubin	0.1–0.5 mg/dl
Serum calcium	8.7–9.1 mg/dl
Serum phosphorus	5–6 mg/dl
Alanine aminotransferase (ALT)	37–111 IU/L
Aspartate aminotransferase (AST)	7–151 IU/L
Alkaline phosphatase	152–212 IU/L
Creatinine phosphokinase	455–551 IU/L

Sulfadimethoxine is recommended for treatment of coccidia, while metronidazole is the drug of choice for *Giardia* spp. infections.

THERAPEUTICS AND SURGICAL CONSIDERATIONS

The most effective route to administer fluids to sick sugar gliders is via an intraosseous catheter. A 24-gauge intraosseous catheter should be placed in the proximal tibia with up to 10% of the patient's body weight in the appropriate fluids administered.[1]

Sugar gliders are small animals and all precautions used for other animals of their size should be taken into consideration prior, during, and after surgery. The surgical candidate should be fasted for 4 hours prior to the initiation of the procedure.[1] Care in providing external heat, hemostasis, and fluid therapy during surgery is essential for a successful completion and an uneventful recovery.

DISEASES

This section will review the common sugar glider diseases seen in veterinary practice. An overview of etiology, treatment, and prevention will follow a brief description of the disease presentation.

NUTRITIONAL OSTEODYSTROPHY

The most common disease seen in captive-bred sugar gliders is nutritional osteodystrophy.[1] Animals that present with severe depression and hind limb paralysis will radiographically reveal osteoporosis and pathologic fractures.[1] Treatment consists of cage rest, supplemental calcium and vitamin D_3, and diet modification.[1] A preventive diet should contain approximately 1% calcium, 0.5% phosphorous, and 1,500 IU/kg vitamin D_3 on a dry-weight basis.[1] Poor nutrition can also lead to obesity, emaciation, and constipation in sugar gliders.

PASTEURELLA MULTOCIDA

Pasteurella multocida has been identified in sugar glider deaths that resulted from generalized organ and subcutaneous abscessation.[1] Prevention starts with keeping the sugar gliders away from rabbits that may be subclinical carriers of this bacterial organism. The treatment of choice is enrofloxicin.

REFERENCES

1. Pye, G. and Carpenter, J.W. "A Guide to Medicine and Surgery in Sugar Gliders." *Vet Medicine*, (October 1999): 891–904.

2. Ness, R.D. "Clinical Pathology and Sample Collection of Exotic Small Mammals." *Vet Clinics of North America (Exotic Animal Practice)* 2, no. 3 (1999): 591–620.

CHAPTER 8

FISH

INTRODUCTION

The popularity of ornamental fish dates back over 2,000 years in China. In the United States, interest in ornamental fish rose during the 1940s with the advent of aviation and the importation of fish from around the world. The advancement of aquarium technologies, such as filtration and nutrition, has enabled this hobby to continue to flourish today.

Most ornamental fish are maintained in aquariums within the home, although the popularity of outdoor ponds continues to rise. Historically, ornamental fish were considered replaceable pets; however, as the value of these animals has risen, pet owners have sought the advice of veterinary professionals to manage their valuable collections. With the improvement of life-support systems, such as filters, fish are living longer, with some cyprinids, such as the goldfish, living well over 10–20 years. As these animals live longer and owners become attached to their pets, veterinarians and their technicians will be expected to give the same high quality care that they provide for other domestic species.

ANATOMY

A basic understanding of anatomy should be developed prior to working with an animal species. A background knowledge of anatomy will prove beneficial when collecting diagnostic samples or administering therapeutics. The focus of this chapter will be on teleosts or boney fishes.

Fish are covered with a mucous coat that is produced by cells in their integument. This mucous coat serves as the first line of defense against pathogenic organisms, such as bacteria, fungi, and viruses. The mucous barrier contains various sized proteins (e.g., immunoglobulins) that bind these pathogens and prevent invasion. If this protective barrier is penetrated, fish have little protection against many of these pathogens once they penetrate the integument. Fish should be handled only when necessary to prevent damaging this protective barrier.

The scales of a fish are located in the dermis and provide protection over the musculature. There are several types of scale found on the teleosts including ganoid, cycloid, and ctenoid. The ganoid and cycloid scales are found on the more primitive species of teleosts, whereas the ctenoid scales are found on the more evolutionary advanced fish. The scales serve as a protective armor and damage or loss of the scales may result in the introduction of opportunistic infections. Handling should be minimized to avoid traumatizing the scales.

Teleosts typically have two sets of paired fins, the pectoral and pelvic fins, and three unpaired fins: the dorsal, anal, and caudal fins. Fins are used for steering, balancing, and braking. Certain species have modified fins to adapt to certain niches. For example, the anal fin of the knifefish is a large single fin located on the ventrum of the animal and serves as the primary source of locomotion. Spines may be associated with some fins and serve as a defense mechanism. The lionfish (*Pterois volitans*) produces venom that can be injected into a potential predator, causing significant pain and discomfort. Knowledge of the species that produce venom is essential to prevent injury to the handler. Fish may damage their spines when captured in a net. To prevent this, fish may be scooped into a plastic cup or bucket to facilitate removal from an aquarium.

Gills are the primary respiratory organs of most fish, although certain species use accessory organs to aid in the absorption of oxygen. Gills serve to absorb oxygen, excrete waste products (e.g., ammonia and carbon dioxide) and regulate ion and water balance. Teleosts have four pairs of gills. The gills are attached to a boney gill arch and each gill is comprised of primary and secondary lamellae. The secondary lamella is the site of gas exchange. Exposure to parasites and toxic compounds, such as ammonia, results in the excessive production of mucus, which can impede gas exchange. Affected animals present with rapid opercular movements, or gulping for air at the surface of the water, and may die suddenly.

Fish possess a two-chambered heart: a single atrium and ventricle. The heart is located ventral to the pharynx and cranial to the liver. Unoxygenated blood is pumped from the heart to the gills where it is oxygenated and distributed to the rest of the body. Fish possess two portal systems, a renal portal system that drains the caudal musculature and a hepatic portal system that drains venous blood from the digestive tract.

The lateral line is a mechanosensory structure that is used by fish to monitor changes in sound waves and water pressure. The lateral line originates on the head, around the eyes and nares, and extends along the lateral body wall. Certain groups of marine fish, including tangs and angelfish, maintained in captivity may develop head and lateral line erosions. The specific etiologies for this syndrome have not been elucidated, but dietary deficiency, water quality, and infectious diseases are all suspected.

The digestive tracts of fish vary depending on their feeding strategy. The length of a herbivore's digestive tract is much longer than that of an omnivore or a carnivore. The stomach is absent in some species, such as the goldfish and carp. Pyloric cecae are found in some species of fish, which secrete digestive enzymes and increase the absorptive surface area of the digestive tract. The number of pyloric cecae may be used in fish identification to differentiate certain species. Fish possess a large liver that is located in the cranial area of the body cavity. The normal color of the liver should be red-brown; however, yellow, fatty livers are a common finding at necropsy. This finding is often the result of diets rich in fats and protein.

Fish possess a single kidney that is divided into an anterior and posterior segment. The kidney is located retroperitoneally in the dorsal body wall. The kidney functions primarily as an osmoregulatory and hematopoietic organ. The anterior kidney and the interstitium of the posterior segment serve as the primary sites for blood cell and immunoglobulin production; fish do not possess bone marrow. The posterior kidney primarily regulates electrolyte and urine output. Fish that are found in a saltwater, or hypertonic environment, tend to lose water and absorb salts. To prevent dehydration, these fish must drink water and excrete excess electrolytes, such as sodium and chloride, through the kidney and gills. Fish that live in a freshwater, or hypotonic environment, constantly absorb water by osmosis. To prevent over-hydration, freshwater fish excrete large volumes of dilute urine.

Fish possess a defense mechanism—composed of free and fixed phagocytic macrophages located in the spleen, heart, and kidney—which filters foreign material from the blood. The erythrocytes of fish are oval-shaped with a pale cytoplasm and a centrally located nucleus. Fish leukocytes may be divided into two groups: agranular and granular. Agranular leukocytes include the thrombocyte, lymphocyte, and monocyte, whereas the granular leukocytes include the neutrophil and eosinophil. Thrombocytes have a small nucleus and a spindle-shaped cell. These cells are analogous to platelets in mammals and are responsible for blood clotting. Lymphocytes are the most common cell type in fish and are morphologically similar to those in mammals. Monocytes are the largest leukocyte and have a pale blue-gray cytoplasm. Neutrophils possess rod-shaped granules and are weakly phagocytic. Eosinophils exist in some species of fish, but their function is unclear. The existence of basophils is controversial.

HUSBANDRY

AQUARIUM

Fish are primarily housed in a glass or acrylic tank. The primary differences between these tanks are that glass weighs more than acrylic, acrylic scratches more easily, and acrylic tanks are available in a wider range of sizes. Acrylic tanks are popular with marine fish enthusiasts. Tanks come in a wide range of sizes and shapes. Recommendations should be based on the type of fish an individual expects to maintain and the aesthetic appeal of the aquarium as a piece of furniture. For example, freshwater angelfish should be maintained in a deep aquarium to prevent cramping of their tall dorsal and anal fins.

Water weighs approximately eight pounds per gallon. The weight of a large aquarium can place significant stresses on a floor. A pet owner should assess the structural integrity of a floor prior to placing a large aquarium in the home. An aquarium should be placed on a secure, level stand.

Most fish are ectotherms, or "cold-blooded," and are dependent on their environmental temperature to regulate their core body temperature. To maintain the overall health of these animals they should be provided a constant environmental temperature. A commercially available aquarium heater can be used to establish an appropriate temperature. Freshwater tropical species should be provided a water temperature between 76–78°F. Certain species (e.g., Discus: *Symphosodon aquafasciatus*) may require higher temperatures (80–82°F) to stimulate their reproductive cycle. Freshwater cold-water species (e.g., goldfish and koi) should be maintained between 65–68°F. Marine tropical species tolerate temperatures between 74–78°F. Fish that are maintained at low temperatures will develop hypothermia and be susceptible to chronic infections. Fish maintained at excessive temperatures often become hyperthermic and die. Outdoor pond fish may develop hyperthermia in certain climates and should be provided appropriate shade.

NUTRITION

There are a variety of commercially available fish foods in the pet retail trade (Figure 8-1). Many of these diets are specifically formulated to meet the needs of specific animals, including herbivores, omnivores, and carnivores. Commercial fish foods are sold in flake and pelleted rations. In certain fish, especially ornamental

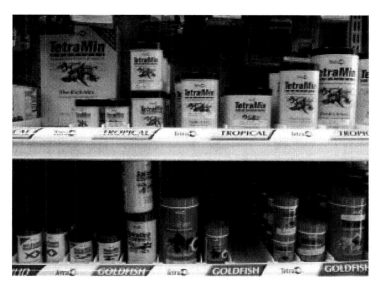

Figure 8-1 Fish food. A variety of food used for fish maintained in hobby aquariums is shown here.

goldfish, the ingestion of floating pellets has been associated with buoyancy problems. Fish that develop these problems should be offered sinking pellets. Obesity is a common problem identified in captive ornamental fish because of a combination of high-fat commercial diets and restricted exercise (aquarium size). Restricted feeding and providing the largest swimming area possible will reduce the potentially life-threatening problems associated with obesity. Live foods are routinely offered to carnivorous fish to balance commercial food preparations and to increase exercise levels. Live foods may transmit disease and should only be purchased through a reputable dealer.

FILTRATION

In nature, waste products produced by fish, plants, and other sources are carried away by flowing water, reducing the potential dangers to fish. In the home aquarium, wastes and toxins can accumulate, leading to a dangerous situation for fish. Filtration is the key to maintaining "healthy" water for fish in an aquarium or pond. There are three primary types of filtration currently used, including mechanical, biologic, and chemical. The different types of filtration work independently of one another and can be used in combination.

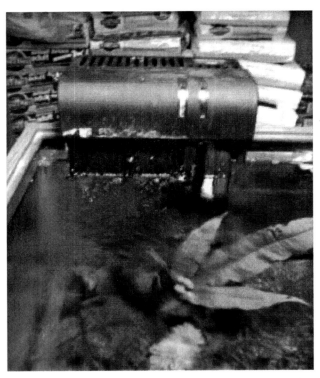

Figure 8-2 Power filter. This is a typical external filter used in hobby fish aquariums.

Mechanical Filtration

Mechanical filtration removes organic debris from the water by passing it through a filter material, such as floss, fiber, or a paper cartridge. The amount of work that this type of filter can perform depends on the type and size of the filter material and the motor or pump that is moving the water past the filter material

(Figure 8-2). A densely packed fiber or small pore size in the paper cartridge will restrict the size of waste that can pass. Maintenance of these filters involves cleaning or replacement of the floss or cartridge. The air pressure exerted by the pump will also affect a mechanical filter. The faster the pump pushes water past the filter material, the quicker it will clog. Mechanical filtration is very useful in both the home aquarium and outdoor pond. This type of filtration is best used with other types of filtration (chemical and biological) to improve the overall quality of water in the system. Mechanical filtration should always be used with a sand filter or bead filter. The mechanical filter will protect the sand or bead filter by removing large particulate matter, which might otherwise clog the biologic filter. Mechanical filtration does have limitations and is not effective in trapping finite particles or chemicals.

Biologic Filtration

Biologic filtration is essential for the removal of toxic compounds, such as ammonia and nitrite. Biologic filtration is the most common type of filtration used in the home aquarium and outdoor pond. There are many different types of biologic filtration, including undergravel filters, bio-wheels, sand or bead filters, and wet-dry filters. A biologic filter should be selected based upon the size of the aquarium (gallons of water), number of fish (density), and frequency of feeding.

Nitrogen is a component of protein. When fish are fed, they take the protein and convert it to energy and waste product. The waste product is converted into ammonia and excreted from both the gills and urine. In an aquarium, ammonia levels can build to dangerous levels for fish, leading to illness or death. Ammonia is an irritant to the gills and skin of fish. Fish suffering from ammonia toxicity may become tachypneic, gasp at the surface, try to jump out of the aquarium, or rub against rocks and plants.

Total ammonia-nitrogen (TAN) is divided into two forms, ionized (NH_4^+) and un-ionized (NH_3). The un-ionized form is toxic, while the ionized form is considered safe. The quantity and form of ammonia found in water is dependent upon biologic, chemical, and physical factors. Biologic factors include the number of fish, amount of food offered, live plants, etc. The chemical factors include pH and alkalinity. When the pH is low or acidic, the majority of ammonia in the water is ionized or nontoxic; whereas, when the pH is high or basic, the un-ionized or toxic form is more common.

Remember, even at an acid pH, enough toxic ammonia (un-ionized) can be present to cause problems for fish. A physical factor that affects the amount of the toxic form of ammonia in the water is temperature. As water temperature increases, the amount of ionized or toxic ammonia also increases.

There are several factors that can affect the function of a biologic filter, including temperature, oxygen content, and drugs/therapeutics. In outdoor ponds when the water temperature drops below 65°F, nitrite is not converted into nitrate as rapidly because the *Nitrobacter* bacteria do not tolerate the cold. During those times when the water temperature may drop, closely monitor nitrite and nitrate levels. To prevent excess work on the biologic filter, stop or reduce the amount of food being offered to the fish. Both of the bacteria essential to the biologic filter need oxygen. In the home aquarium, oxygen levels are often adequate; however, in outdoor ponds oxygen levels can become depleted, depending on the time of day or season. (See the oxygen section.) To prevent a problem with oxygen depletion, aerate the water with a fountain or air stone during the times when a problem might occur.

A biologic filter requires time to become established. The amount of time depends upon the temperature of the water and the organic load on the system. For example, a system maintained at 23°C takes 4–6 weeks to become established. Commercial microbial products are available that claim to expedite the establishment of the microflora. Unfortunately, there is no hard evidence to support this theory. Water samples, filter pads, or aquarium substrates from established systems have also been used to seed a tank. The addition of these products may lead to the introduction of potential pathogens.

Chemical Filtration

There are a number of different types of chemical filters available in the pet trade. Chemical filtration refers to those filters that remove toxic compounds by binding them or converting them into nontoxic substances. The original form of chemical filtration was activated carbon. Carbon can bind a number of different substances (nonspecific). When the binding sites are full, they no longer act as filters and need to be replaced or cleaned. Other forms of chemical filtration are more specific, such as the resins that only bind ammonia. There are other forms of chemical filtration such as ultraviolet sterilizers and protein skimmers that alter or trap compounds. Ultraviolet sterilizers expose compounds to short wavelength light, altering their form and rendering them harmless. Protein skimmers trap protein in bubbles so that they can be separated from the water and removed. Chemical filtration, in combination with mechanical and biologic filtration, can improve the water quality dramatically, creating a "healthy" environment for fish.

Ultraviolet (UV) sterilizers can be used to control certain pathogens and algae. A UV sterilizer has a UV bulb encased in a waterproof sheath within a cylinder. As water passes through the cylinder, the water is exposed to ultraviolet light, which can alter the DNA or RNA of a microorganism. The amount of time that it takes for the water to pass the bulb and the bulb wattage determine the effectiveness of the UV sterilizer. A low wattage bulb in a short cylinder will have little effect on pathogens. These systems have also been used with great success at controlling pathogens and algae in outdoor ponds.

WATER QUALITY

Water quality is very important to the health of a fish, and poor water quality can prove fatal. There are two types of systems that can be used: open and closed. In open water systems, the water in the aquarium is continually replenished using a fresh water source. An individual who lives by the ocean may collect seawater for a home marine aquarium, although this is not recommended because of the potential contaminants in the water. Open water systems are rarely used because they are labor-intensive and require regular exchange of the entire system. The majority of home aquariums utilize closed recirculating systems, which recirculate the same water over and over again using a filter. In the closed system, fresh water is added only after evaporation or at the time of a water change.

Ammonia, Nitrite, and Nitrate

Ammonia is produced in fish as an end product of protein catabolism and is excreted directly across the gills into the aquatic medium. Ammonia is also derived from feces, uneaten food, and decaying organic matter. Ammonia nitrogen can occur in two forms: ammonium (NH_4^+) and ammonia (NH_3). Ammonia is the more toxic form to fish.[1] The relative concentration of each form varies with water pH and temperature.[2]

Ammonia is soluble in water and minimal amounts are lost through evaporation. In a closed system, such as an aquarium or backyard pond, ammonia levels can build up to toxic quantities (>1 ppm). Even low levels of ammonia can be toxic to the gills and skin, resulting in increased susceptibility to infections. Fish suffering from ammonia toxicity appear irritated, gasp at the water surface, and may rub against rocks in the enclosure as a result of the irritation caused by the toxin. Ammonia levels should be monitored closely in new systems or systems that contain a large number of fish. Ammonia should be tested weekly using a standardized commercial test kit, which is available at local pet retailers. In an established system, ammonia levels should be zero. If the ammonia levels begin to rise, then the system should be reevaluated. Overfeeding and overstocking an aquarium can overburden the biologic filter. Severe temperature fluctuations and insufficient oxygen levels may also result in a significant loss of the biological filter. This is especially common in ponds that have significant summer algal blooms. New systems require time to become established, and new fish should be added gradually to prevent an overload of the biological filter.

Since ammonia is a common waste product produced by fish and excessive decaying food, most problems can be prevented by limiting the stocking numbers in an aquarium and by offering only the quantity of food that the fish will consume within a 2–5 minute period. In cases where ammonia levels are creating problems, the first recommendation is to remove 25–50% of the water from the system and replace it with fresh, dechlorinated water. There are commercial products available that can chelate the ammonia source, but they are only a temporary solution. The primary cause of the elevated ammonia levels must be diagnosed and corrected.

Ammonia is a colorless, odorless substance that can cause significant mortalities in a home aquarium. Most inexperienced aquarists tend to single-out infectious diseases when they experience fish losses; however, poor water quality (e.g., excessive ammonia or nitrite) is often a primary or secondary cause of mortalities in these animals and should be tested on a regular basis.

The nitrogen cycle eliminates ammonia by converting it to less toxic compounds. Ammonia is initially oxidized to nitrite (NO_2^-) by bacteria (*Nitrosomonas* spp.) within the aquatic system. Nitrite is also toxic to fish and can be rapidly absorbed across the gills. Affected animals develop a methemoglobinemia and have a characteristic "brown-blood," gasp for air at the water surface, and die suddenly. Nitrite levels in an aquatic system may rise soon after treatment of the water with antibacterial compounds or a reduction in water temperature. Antibiotics added to the water are nonselective and will kill both pathogenic and commensal organisms. These compounds may kill enough bacteria associated with the biologic filter to prevent the oxidation of ammonia and nitrite. *Nitrosomonas* spp. will recolonize before *Nitrobacter* spp., so ammonia levels should be expected to decrease before nitrites. *Nitrobacter* spp. are more sensitive to temperature fluctuations than *Nitrosomonas* spp., therefore, elevated nitrite levels are often detected soon after a reduction in water temperature. Nitrite levels less than 0.5 ppm are generally regarded as safe; levels less than 3.0 ppm are associated with stress and may predispose fish to opportunistic infections; levels greater than 5 ppm are considered toxic.

When fish show clinical signs associated with nitrite toxicity, they should be removed from the toxic water and placed into a fresh, dechlorinated, well-oxygenated system. (Fish with methemoglobinemia have a reduced oxygen carrying capacity and require well-oxygenated water.) This can be accomplished by placing into a hospital tank a fine-mist airstone that creates a break in the water surface tension, increasing water oxygen levels. A significant water change (25–50%) should be made in the original aquarium or pond and the biologic filter reestablished.

In the nitrogen cycle, nitrite is further oxidized to nitrate (NO_3^-) by *Nitrobacter* spp. Reports of nitrate toxicity are rare in fresh and saltwater fish, but elevated levels may be stressful and predispose the animals to opportunistic pathogens. Nitrate is utilized by plants and algae as a food source. Nitrate can be removed from an aquatic system by performing regular water changes.

"New Tank" Syndrome

"New tank" syndrome is a common problem reported by beginner/novice aquarists who overload a newly established biologic filter. "New tank" syndrome primarily occurs when fish are overstocked in a new aquarium. The high density of fish creates a high ammonia load on the new system. This is often coupled with over-feeding, which leads to an additional organic load on the system and a rise in ammonia levels. In most cases, the owners report acute death of the fish and the clinical signs are consistent with ammonia and nitrite toxicity. These problems can be prevented if the new owner is patient and realizes the importance of providing a break-in period for the filter (4–6 weeks). Fish should be stocked gradually, usually 1–2 fish per week. A standard rule of thumb for a freshwater stocking density is 1–1.5 inches of fish per gallon of water, whereas in saltwater systems the stocking density should be 2–2.5 inches of fish per gallon of water. With the advent of new filtration systems, stocking densities will continue to increase; however, if the filter becomes compromised or fails, the results would be disastrous.

Oxygen

Fish acquire free oxygen directly from the water. Oxygen diffuses into water at the surface when the surface tension of the water is broken. The amount of available or dissolved oxygen (DO) within the system can be measured using special equipment. In most cases, a DO >5 ppm is sufficient to maintain fish. In most home aquariums, there is sufficient DO.

Oxygen depletion is a major concern in outdoor ponds during the summer months. During the day, plants produce their own food (photosynthesis) by taking carbon dioxide from the water and using energy produced by the sun. As plants make their food, they release oxygen into the water. During the night when plants or algae cannot undergo photosynthesis, they actually consume oxygen. In ponds with a large number of plants or algae, the oxygen levels in the water can fall to dangerously low levels for the fish. Another factor that may affect oxygen levels in water is temperature. Oxygen is lost to the atmosphere more rapidly in warm water than cold water. The use of aerators or fountains, especially at night, will help maintain adequate levels of oxygen in a pond.

Water pH

The pH of water is calculated as the negative logarithm of hydrogen ions. In simplest terms, pH can be divided into 3 categories: acid, neutral, and basic. The range of pH values fits on a scale of 1–14. Values below 7.0 represent acidic water, values between 7.0–7.9 are neutral, and values above 8.0 are basic. The pH in most aquariums and ponds should fall between 6.5–8.5. In the extreme ranges (<4 or >10), water would be so acidic or basic that it would burn the fish. This means that the difference between 7.0 and 8.0 is much more significant than you might expect, since the pH values are based on a logarithmic scale. Therefore, if the pH is allowed to fluctuate, fish will become stressed and more susceptible to disease.

The pH of natural bodies of water varies based on the substrate, water shed, and other environmental factors. Fish from Central and South America thrive in water that is neutral or slightly acidic, whereas fish from Africa and Asia thrive better at neutral to alkaline water.

Water should always be tested prior to replacement into an aquarium. There are a number of factors that may affect the pH in an aquarium or pond, including the biologic filter, fish density, vegetation, and algae. Biologic filtration actually produces acid when ammonia is converted into nitrite. If the water has a low buffering capacity and the aquarium or pond biologic filter is converting a large amount of ammonia, the pH could become very acidic. Fish produce carbon dioxide (CO_2) as a waste product. When an aquarium or pond is heavily stocked with fish, the amount of CO_2 can build up in the water. Carbon dioxide promotes acid production and can actually decrease the pH (acidic). Plants and algae, which use photosynthesis during the day to make energy, utilize CO_2. However, at night, plants and algae utilize oxygen (like fish) and expel CO_2 as a waste product. In a system with a large amount of plants and algae, the pH can drop to a dangerously low level. Fish die-offs in ponds are often associated with high CO_2, low pH, and low oxygen levels. When plants or fish die, they also release compounds that can lower the pH. To prevent this from becoming a problem, always remove dead fish or plants immediately.

Chlorine

Chlorine is a gas that is added to our municipal water supplies to protect us from bacteria and other harmful organisms. Unfortunately, chlorine is toxic to fish. When a fish is placed in chlorinated water, the chlorine crosses the gills and blocks the fish's ability to absorb oxygen, which causes suffocation. This whole process can take minutes to hours, depending upon the amount of chlorine in the water. Sodium thiosulfate can be added to tap water to neutralize chlorine, immediately making the water safe for fish. Municipal water supplies add variable amounts of chlorine at different times of the year, depending upon the source of water. If you have questions about the timing or the amounts of chlorine that are being added, call your local water company. Always test the water before replacing it in the aquarium or pond to ensure that the chlorine has been removed.

Chloramine

Chloramines are also routinely added to municipal water supplies for sterilization purposes. Chloramines are formed by combining chlorine with ammonia. Commercial dechlorinators may be added to tap water to neutralize chlorine; however, the ammonia will remain in the water. Ammonia is toxic to fish and can prove fatal to fish at levels higher than (1 ppm). A functional biologic filter will convert the ammonia to nitrate.

Hardness

Hardness measures the amount of divalent cations, primarily calcium and magnesium, in the water. In natural waters, the divalent ions are derived from limestone, salts, and soils. The normal range for hardness in freshwater systems is 0–250 mg/L, whereas in saltwater systems the total hardness can exceed 10,000 mg/L.[3] Calcium and magnesium play an intricate role in water quality conditions. Calcium appears to protect fish that are exposed to a low pH or elevated ammonia by altering osmoregulatory functions.[3] Calcium and magnesium are essential to growth and development of fish fry.[4] Calcium and magnesium can also protect fish from heavy metal exposure by competing for gill absorption sites. Copper is routinely used to treat parasites. Calcium and magnesium will compete with the copper for absorption sites, reducing the effectiveness of the copper. Distilled water should never be used to replenish water in an aquarium because it is deficient in these essential cations.

Alkalinity

In natural water systems, such as lakes, fish are exposed to a relatively stable pH because of buffers. The most common buffers in aquatic systems are bicarbonate (HCO_3) and carbonate (CO_3^{2-}). Other buffers that may occur in water in lesser amounts include: hydroxide (OH-), silicates, phosphates, and borates. The quantity of buffers within a system depends upon location. Some municipal water supplies contain minuscule amounts of buffers, while others may have large quantities of buffers. There are commercial buffers that can be added to an aquarium or pond to increase the total alkalinity in the system, creating a more stable pH.

Total alkalinity also plays a role in the chemistry of potential toxins such as lead, zinc, and copper. Heavy metals are absorbed from the water by the gills and are fatal to fish.

Bicarbonate and carbonate can actually bind the heavy metals, rendering them harmless. This is important to remember when treating fish with nonchelated copper. If the alkalinity is high, the unchelated copper may be bound and rendered useless.

Monitoring Water Quality

New Tanks: Water should be tested weekly for ammonia, nitrite, nitrate, pH, alkalinity, and hardness. If problems occur, test water more frequently. Allow 4–6 weeks for the biologic filter to become established. Add only one or two fish at a time so that the biologic filter is not overloaded. Always test new water for the previously mentioned parameters and for chlorine and chloramine before replacing it in the aquarium or pond.

Established Tanks: Replace 10–20% of the water every 1–3 weeks. The frequency of water change will depend on the load on the system (i.e., size of aquarium, number of fish, amount of food offered). A small aquarium will need more frequent changes than a large aquarium. By closely monitoring the water (ammonia, nitrite, nitrate, pH, alkalinity, and hardness), you will be able to determine when the water will need to be changed. Before replacing the water, be sure to test it for the same parameters, as well as chlorine and chloramine.

TRANSPORT TO THE VETERINARY HOSPITAL

Fish should be transported in a plastic, sealed container. The container should be used exclusively to transport fish and never reused to carry human food items. The container should be cleaned with warm, soapy water and rinsed thoroughly after each use. Bleach should never be used to clean the container. The water used to transport the animal should come from the home aquarium. A separate container of aquarium water should also be brought to the veterinary hospital—in case of spillage and for water quality testing. The fish should be transported immediately to the veterinary hospital. Special precautions should be made during the winter and summer to prevent water temperature fluctuations, such as pre-heating or cooling the transport automobile in the winter and summer respectively. Signs of transport stress may not be apparent for several days after the move, so animals should be monitored closely for 3–5 days post-transport.[5]

HISTORY

A thorough history is key to developing a diagnostic and therapeutic plan. There are four key areas that must be addressed in the history: the owner's general knowledge, the aquarium environment, the water, and the fish. Questions regarding the owner's general knowledge of aquarium management should include the length of ownership, if there are multiple aquaria, where the fish were obtained, the time spent viewing the fish, and the weekly maintenance program. The history of the aquarium environment should include questions about tank volume, tank placement, tank top, lighting, heating, filtration, substrate, and aquarium decorations (e.g., plants, rocks, logs, and toys). Tank volume is important because it allows the veterinary technician to determine the relative stocking density of the aquarium. The placement of the tank within the home may provide insight into problems associated with algal overgrowth (e.g., direct sunlight exposure) or toxins (e.g., cleaning sprays). Some fish owners do not cover their aquariums with a top. Tanks without tops experience faster evaporation and are more prone to fish losses because of jumping. There are a number of different lighting systems available for the home aquarium. Owners should be asked whether they have fluorescent or incandescent lighting, the bulb wattage, and the amount of time the lighting remains on during the day. Incandescent lights exert radiant heat and are associated with increased water temperatures. Fluorescent lighting, especially full-spectrum lighting, is preferred for live aquatic plant systems. Most aquaria are heated with thermostatically controlled heaters. Questions regarding heater usage (yes or no), type, and wattage size should be asked. Owners should also be asked if they use a thermometer and, if so, the temperature in the aquarium. Fish are poikilotherms and must be provided an appropriate environmental temperature. Because there are a number of different types of filters, questions should be asked to determine the types of filters, length of usage, and the owner's general knowledge of filtration. Information should be ascertained regarding the aquarium decorations, such as plants, rocks, logs, and toys. The addition of new live plants may serve as an introduction of disease.

Most aquarium clients have a limited knowledge of water chemistry; therefore, veterinary technicians must be patient with their clients when taking a history on the water quality. Questions must be asked regarding the source of the water, the frequency that the water is changed, and the water quality tests that have been performed. Veterinary hospitals that work with ornamental fish should have water quality test kits and should perform the appropriate water tests during the visit (Figure 8-3).

The final history questions should focus on the fish. Questions regarding types of fish, number of fish, and length of ownership are all important. Many infectious disease cases are the direct result of adding new, unquarantined fish. The types of other aquatic organisms, such as snails, must also be addressed as these animals may also introduce disease. Owners should be asked whether the fish are eating and if any abnormal behaviors have been noted, such as whirling, inverted swimming, jumping, increased breathing, or lethargy. The final questions should address the number of affected fish, specific lesions, and the duration of the presenting disease.

PHYSICAL EXAMINATION

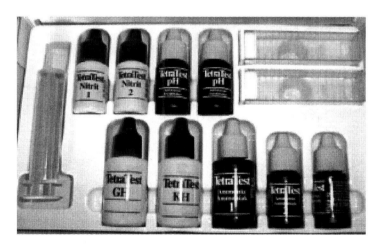

Figure 8-3 Test kit. Kits such as the one shown here are needed to determine and maintain water quality in aquariums.

There are two parts to a fish physical examination: the hands-off and the hands-on. Fish should always be observed from a distance prior to handling. Observe the fish for abnormalities in behavior, breathing, and attitude. Any abnormal findings should be recorded prior to a hands-on examination.

A fish may be captured with a net or a gloved hand, or it may be scooped into a plastic cup or bucket. Animals in a large aquarium must be caught with a net. Netting a fish can be a very traumatic experience. It is best to reduce the lighting in the room when capturing a fish to prevent it from swimming into the tank walls and injuring itself. Once the fish is captured, it should be transferred into a bucket with water collected from the primary aquarium.

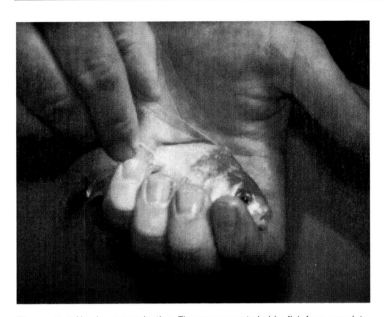

Figure 8-4 Hands-on examination. The proper way to hold a fish for a complete physical exam is shown here.

A hands-on physical examination of a fish should be performed in a thorough and rapid manner (Figure 8-4). Generally, a fish is anesthetized for a physical examination and diagnostic tests are collected at the same time. Tricaine methane sulfonate is the anesthetic of choice. The physical examination should be performed out of water to improve visualization of the animal. The fish should be replaced into the water bucket every 30–45 seconds during the procedure to allow it to respire. The fish should be cupped in the hand with minimal restraint, as the protective mucous layer and scales may be damaged from minor manipulation. Although the examination may be performed in moist, bare hands, moistened latex gloves are preferred.

Handlers should have a basic knowledge of the fish that they are working with to prevent injury to themselves and other hospital staff. Many ornamental fish have spines associated with their fins, which can cause pain upon puncture and become a source of infection to the handler. There are also a number of venomous ornamental fish, such as the lionfish, which can inject venom; they should only be handled by professionals. In most cases, anesthetizing fish is preferred to ensure safety to the animals and the handler.

SURGICAL AND ANESTHETIC ASSISTANCE

SURGERY

Surgical procedures are becoming more routine in fish. The basic tenets of surgery in domestic species apply to fish surgery, too. Fish surgery can be performed in or out of water. The preferred method is out of water because it increases visualization of the surgical field. Tricaine methane sulfonate is the anesthetic of choice for surgical procedures. Surgical procedures should be performed using a recirculating anesthetic machine. Preparation of the surgical area should be performed with a non-insulting disinfectant or saline. Avoid alcohol rinses for surgical preparation because it increases heat loss. Many disinfectants cause chemical burns or are toxic and should be avoided. Microsurgical equipment should be used to perform surgical procedures in fish.

ANESTHESIA

Historically, veterinarians working with lower vertebrates (e.g., fish, amphibians, and reptiles) have relied on "bruticaine" to restrain animals for physical examination and short surgical procedures. This technique is unacceptable, as there are a number of safe, reliable anesthetic agents that can be used to appropriately restrain or anesthetize a fish for different procedures.

A fish should be thoroughly evaluated prior to performing an anesthetic procedure. Fish that are stressed, maintained under inappropriate water temperatures, or have ingested a recent meal are not considered good anesthetic candidates. Prospective anesthetic candidates should be maintained in clean, dechlorinated, well-oxygenated water (5–10 ppm) under reduced lighting. Food should be withheld for a minimum of 12 hours to ensure that they do not regurgitate and contaminate the anesthetic solution.

Always wear a pair of latex gloves when handling fish to administer an anesthetic (e.g., intramuscular injection) or to perform a procedure. Fish that are mishandled may develop an injury to their integument, damaging their dermis (scale-loss), and increasing their susceptibility to opportunistic pathogens. Gloves are also beneficial to handlers and will protect them from potentially zoonotic diseases such as *Mycobacterium* spp.

Monitoring fish during an anesthetic procedure can be difficult. In most cases, opercular movement, loss of equilibrium, sensitivity to painful stimuli, fin color, and gill color are used to assess the patient. In larger specimens, a pulse oximeter, ECG, or crystal doppler may be used to monitor heart rate, although the heart of a fish may continue to pump for a period of time after the animal is dead. In the case of waterborne anesthetics, dechlorinated water may be used to irrigate the gills and "lighten" the plane of anesthesia.

The most widely used anesthetic agent for fish is tricaine methane sulfonate (MS-222). It is a benzocaine derivative with a sulfonate radical. Tricaine methane sulfonate is absorbed across the gill epithelium and biotransformed in the liver and possibly the kidney.[6] The drug and its metabolites are excreted primarily through the gills. The stock solutions are very acidic and should be buffered prior to being used. Tricaine methane sulfonate administered at a 10g/L solution can be used to perform most procedures.[7]

For short procedures (e.g., gill clip), the animal may be removed from the anesthetic tank and resubmerged into the anesthetic solution or recovery tank as needed. For procedures that require a significant time out of water (e.g., surgery), animals should be maintained on a recirculating system. A simple system consisting of an electric submersible pump, flexible tubing, and two reservoirs (1- anesthetic, 1- recovery) may be used to maintain a fish during a surgical procedure. The tubing should be placed directly into the animal's mouth to irrigate the gills. The recirculating pump may be moved from the anesthetic solution to nonanesthetic solution as the anesthetic depth varies.

Quinaldine sulfate is another water-based drug that can be used to anesthetize fish. Quinaldine sulfate, like MS-222, is strongly acidic in solution and should be buffered before use. The dose used for quinaldine sulfate is similar to MS-222, although some consider quinaldine to have a greater margin of safety. Quinaldine is not metabolized by the fish and is excreted unchanged. Quinaldine can be used for many basic procedures, but is not recommended for surgical procedures that require total loss of movement.

Inhalant anesthetics have been used with variable success. An inhalant anesthetic, such as isoflurane, can be poured directly into the aquatic medium in the concentrated form or "aerated" in the form of a gas. Regulating the concentration of anesthetic in the water can be difficult. Incomplete distribution of the inhalant anesthetic in the water column may result in "pockets" of gas and variable anesthetic effects. The use of inhalants places additional risk on individuals performing the surgery; therefore, attempts should be made to scavenge the waste gas.

Reports in lay literature have suggested that carbon dioxide can be used as a fish anesthetic.[8] There are many different commercially available sources of CO_2, including Alka-Seltzer®, carbon dioxide gas (used for aquatic plant aquaria), and sodium bicarbonate. Unfortunately, CO_2 is difficult to regulate, and if not monitored closely, will result in a rapid decrease in pH and the death of the fish. With the availability of safe, effective anesthetics, such as MS-222, there is no reason for veterinarians to use CO_2.

Injectable anesthetics are rarely used to anesthetize ornamental fish because high doses of drug are required and incomplete anesthesia is achieved. Injectable anesthetics have proven effective in elasmobranchs, and current research being performed at Louisiana State University indicates that medetomidine and propofol may be used to effectively immobilize elasmobranchs.

DIAGNOSTIC SAMPLING

A gill biopsy can be performed to assess gill status in animals maintained in poor water quality or to diagnose ectoparasites. Fish should be anesthetized for a gill biopsy to provide appropriate sedation and analgesia. Tricaine methane sulfonate (MS-222) can be used to provide appropriate anesthesia. Once a fish is anesthetized, it should be removed from the anesthetic solution using gloved hands and placed onto a dechlorinated, moist paper towel. A pair of fine iris scissors should be inserted under the operculum and gently lifted, enabling the handler to insert his thumb under the operculum to provide direct visualization of the gills (Figure 8-5). Iris scissors should be reinserted under the operculum, and 3–5 gill filaments should be collected. The gill filaments should be placed onto a slide with 0.9% saline and reviewed under a microscope. Once the procedure has been completed, the animal should recover in dechlorinated, fresh water.

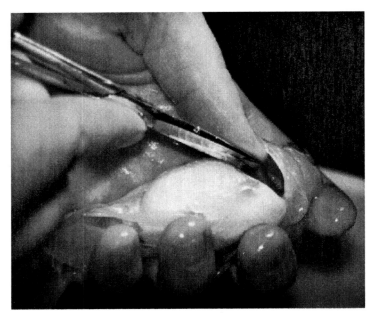

Figure 8-5 Gill biopsy. This is a useful diagnostic tool for identifying diseases associated with the gills.

A skin scrape can be performed to diagnose pathogens on the surface of a fish integument. Once again, the animal should be anesthetized to reduce stress. The animal may be restrained by hand or placed on a moistened paper towel. A microscope slide should be placed on the skin at a 45° angle caudal to the operculum and gently dragged in a caudal direction (Figure 8-6). The fish should recover in dechlorinated water.

A fin biopsy should be performed to evaluate specific lesions on an animal's fins. A fish undergoing this procedure should be anesthetized. A pair of iris scissors should be used to cut a sample of an affected fin between the fin rays (Figure 8-7). The sample should be mixed with 0.9% saline on a microscope slide, covered with a cover slip, and evaluated under a microscope. The fish should be recovered in dechlorinated water.

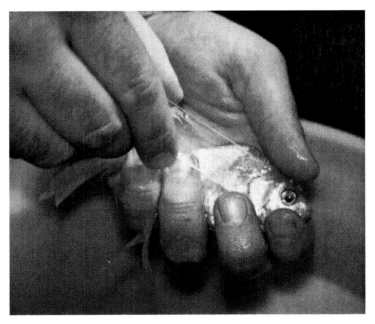

Figure 8-6 Skin scrape. Common skin pathogens are identified through skin scraping and microscopic examination.

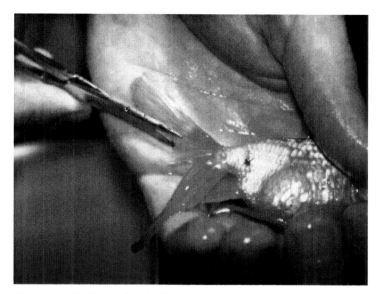

Figure 8-7 Fin biopsy. Certain disease processes may be identified through a fin biopsy.

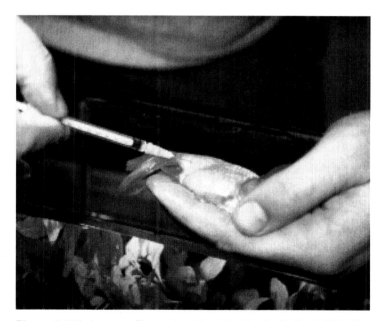

Figure 8-8 Venipuncture. The most useful vein for blood collection in fish is the caudal tail vein.

Fish have evolved to mask their illnesses as a defense mechanism. The examination of blood samples can provide insight into the general health of the animal, which might not otherwise be obvious on physical examination. The volume of blood that can be collected from a fish has been estimated to be similar to mammals, approximately 0.8–1.0% of the body weight.[9] Always pre-load the needle with heparin to prevent blood clotting. The primary site of venipuncture in the fish is the caudal tail vein (Figure 8-8). The caudal tail vein is located ventral to the vertebral column and runs parallel to the spine. A 3-ml syringe with a 25- to 30-gauge needle is recommended for sample collection. The needle should be gently inserted at a 45° angle (between scales) into the caudal peduncle at the level of the lateral line and walked off the ventral edge of the vertebral column until a flash of blood is visualized in the needle. The blood sample from the caudal tail vein can also be collected from a ventral approach. The animal should be held in dorsal recumbency and the needle inserted into the ventral midline of the caudal peduncle at a 90° angle. The needle should be inserted to the level of the vertebral column and gently walked along the spine until a flash of blood is visualized.

MICROBIOLOGY

Microbiologic samples may be collected from a fish during an ante mortem or postmortem exam. Ante mortem samples are routinely collected from specific lesions on the skin, fins, or eyes. Contamination is a significant concern in these cases, and results should be interpreted accordingly. A sterile swab may be rubbed over the affected area to collect the sample. The sample should be refrigerated until it is plated, which should occur within 24 hours.

Postmortem cultures routinely involve internal organs. To ensure sterility, the necropsy should be performed in a consistent manner. Seventy-percent ethyl alcohol should be applied to the ventral surface of the fish and the area flamed. Once the alcohol has burned off, the fish should be opened using sterile scissors and forceps. After the coelomic cavity is exposed, samples can be collected using either a sterile swab or sterile biopsy techniques.

There are many different opinions about the appropriate culture media and incubation temperatures to isolate bacterial pathogens from fish. A standard blood agar plate may be used as the initial plate, or other specialized plates may be used if a specific pathogen is suspected. Salt should be supplemented to the plate when attempting to isolate pathogens from marine fish. Plates should be incubated between 20–25°C. Culture plates should be evaluated for growth at 24- and 48-hour time periods. A Gram-stain should be performed on any isolate. Biochemical identification of the organism should follow standard microbiologic protocol.

RADIOLOGY

There are several case presentations that require radiographic evaluation, including foreign body ingestion, neoplasia, internal abscesses, and swim bladder disease. Fish should be anesthetized during the procedure to prevent thrashing and damage to the mucous

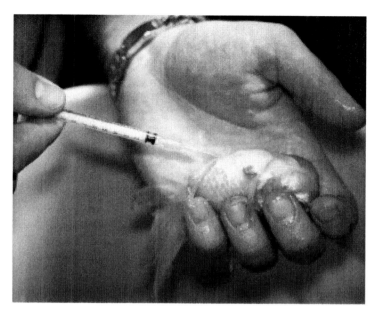

Figure 8-9 Therapeutics. Proper position is shown for intraperitoneal injection.

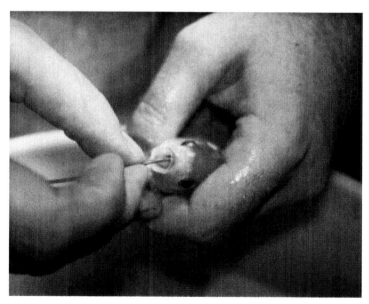

Figure 8-10 Force-feeding. Medication and feeding through a tube is necessary in debilitated fish patients.

barrier and integument. Tricaine methane sulfonate is the anesthetic of choice. The fish should be placed on moistened paper towels during the procedure and recovered as soon as the procedure is completed. The techniques used to perform the radiographs will vary from machine to machine. High-detail films should be used to provide the best radiographic image.

THERAPEUTICS

Therapeutics may be administered to fish in a water bath, per os, intramuscular injection, intraperitoneal injection, or the intravenous route (Figure 8-9). Water bath treatment protocols are of little value to freshwater fish, but have been used with success to treat marine fish. Marine fish actually drink water, so any medication placed in the water will be ingested. Freshwater fish do not drink water and are not likely to receive the same benefit. Carbon filters should be removed when a bath or immersion treatment is used. Per os medications can also be placed into food and delivered to the fish during routine feedings. Unfortunately, many sick fish are anorectic and do not benefit from medicated food. Per os medications can also be administered via a stomach tube (Figure 8-10). A red rubber feeding tube may be used for this procedure. The distance from the mouth to the mid-body should be measured and marked, thereby denoting the approximate location of the stomach. The tube should be inserted to the level of the mark, and the medication delivered. Intramuscular injections are administered into the epaxial muscle surrounding the spine. The needle is inserted between scales. Irritating compounds should not be administered IM because they can lead to muscle necrosis. Intraperitoneal injections are routinely used to administer antibiotics to fish. The fish is held in dorsal recumbency, allowing gravity to drop the viscera, and the injection administered between the scales of the ventrum into the peritoneal cavity (Figure 8-9). Again, insulting compounds should not be used. Intravenous injections are not routinely used, but may be useful during emergency situations. Inappropriate use of antibiotics and antiparasitics may lead to the development of resistant strains of bacteria and parasites.

DISEASES

BACTERIAL DISEASES

Bacterial diseases are commonly reported in ornamental fish. Many of the opportunistic pathogens isolated from sick fish, such as *Aeromonas* spp. and *Pseudomonas* spp., are routinely isolated from the water column. Many of these infections develop when there is damage to the animal's protective integument or immune system. Septicemia is a common finding and must be treated aggressively. The majority of bacterial septicemias are caused by Gram-negative rods. Bacterial infections should be diagnosed by culture and sensitivity. A therapeutic plan should follow the sensitivity results.

VIRAL DISEASES

Viral diseases in ornamental fish are rare. The pathogenicity of viruses can vary with temperature. Most viral infections in fish are host specific. In many cases, young, naive fishes become sick and older animals become carriers. The most commonly reported virus in ornamental fish is lymphocystis, an iridovirus that infects fibroblasts.[10] Affected animals develop large coalescing nodules that can occur anywhere on the body. The virus is self-limiting. In most cases, the fish resolve spontaneously; however, in cases where the lesions affect the eyes or mouth (i.e., its vision or ability to eat), the animal may die. Lymphocystis can be diagnosed on gross examination or histopathology. There is no effective treatment, although the mass may be surgically debulked if the tumor affects the animal's ability to eat, see, or swim.

PARASITES

Parasites are routinely identified on imported ornamental fish. When parasitized animals are added to an established aquarium, the parasites will soon spread to the other tank inhabitants. Both ectoparasites and endoparasites are reported in fish. The clinical signs associated with a parasite infestation will vary depending upon the location of the parasite. Fish with gill flukes (*Dactylogyrids*) will become hypoxic, gulping air at the surface and coughing. Fish infested with skin parasites, such as ich (*Ichthyopthirius multifiliis*), rub against hard surfaces, lose scales, and hemorrhage in the area of parasite attachment (Figure 8-11). Fish with endoparasites are often anorectic, in poor condition, and fail to thrive. The diagnostic tests routinely used to identify ectoparasites include a skin scrape, fin biopsy, and gill clip. A fecal float and direct saline smear should be performed to evaluate endoparasite status.

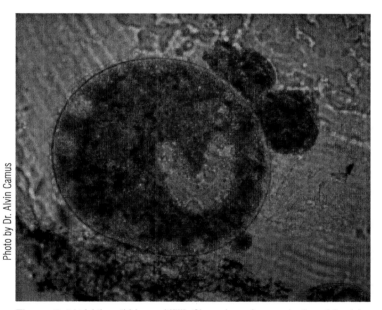

Photo by Dr. Alvin Camus

Figure 8-11 *Ichthyopthirius multifiliis.* Shown is a microscopic view of the *Ich.* organism.

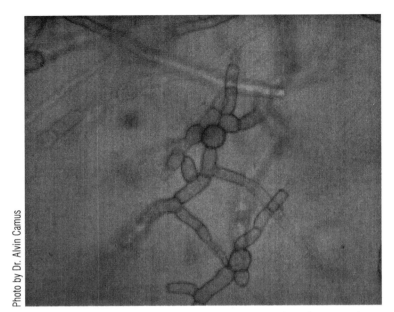

Photo by Dr. Alvin Camus

Figure 8-12 *Saprolegnia.* Shown is a microscopic view of the *Sapro.* organism.

WATER MOLDS

Saprolegnia spp. is a common water mold isolated from tropical ornamental fish and cold-water aquaculture species (Figure 8-12). Water molds are primarily opportunists; they often infect open wounds, although primary infections are also possible. Affected fish generally present with white, cotton-like lesions on fins and skin. A skin scrape or biopsy of an affected area can be used to confirm a diagnosis of water molds, which are classified based on their branching nonseptate hyphae.

ZOONOTIC DISEASES

Humans may be exposed to fishborne diseases through ingestion of contaminated fish or water, or through direct contact with fish or water. Zoonotic diseases attributed to ornamental fish are routinely associated with contamination of open wounds or puncture wounds that occur during handling. Humans with a compromised immune system may be predisposed to opportunistic infections. Most cases of fishborne zoonotic diseases result in mild episodes of the disease.[11] A number of bacteria have been associated with human illness, including: *Clostridium* spp., *Erysipelothrix rhusiopathiae*, *Mycobacterium* spp., *Staphylococcus* spp., and *Streptococcus* spp. Members of the family Enterobacteriaceae, including: *Edwardsiella tarda*, *Klebsiella* spp., *Salmonella* spp., and *Yersinia* spp., are routinely isolated from aquatic environments and have also been associated with human illness. Fish parasites and toxins have been found to cause human illness, but are generally associated with ingestion of the fish. To prevent the transmission of potentially zoonotic diseases, veterinary professionals should follow standard safety protocols and wear protective clothing.

REFERENCES

1. Russo, R.C. "Ammonia, Nitrite, and Nitrate." In Rand, G.M. and Pertocelli, S.R. eds., *Fundamentals of Aquatic Toxicology*. Hemisphere, New York, 1985: 455–471.

2. Emerson, K., Russo, R.C., Lund, R.E., and Thurston, R.V. "Aqueous Ammonia Equilibrium Calculations: Effect of pH and Temperature," *Journal of Fish Research Board of Canada* 32 (1975) 2379–2383.

3. Tucker, C.S. "Water Analysis." In Stoskopf, M.K. ed., *Fish Medicine*. Philadelphia: W.B. Saunders, 1993: 166–197.

4. Piper, R.G., McElwain, J.B., Orne, L.E., McCraren, J.P., Fowler, L.G., and Leonard, J.R. "Fish Hatchery Management." United States Department of Interior, Fish and Wildlife Service, Washington D.C., 1982.

5. Tomasso, J.R., Davis, K.B. and Parker, N.C. "Plasma Corticosteroid and Electrolyte Dynamics of Hybrid Striped Bass (White Bass x Striped Bass) During Netting and Hauling Stress," Proceedings of the World Mariculture Society 11 (1980) 303–310.

6. Allen, J.L. and Hunn, J.B. "Fate and Distribution Studies of Some Drugs Used in Aquaculture," *Veterinary and Human Toxicology* 28 (1986) 21–24.

7. Stoskopf, M.K: "Anesthesia of Pet Fishes." In Bonagura, J.D. ed., *Kirk's Current Veterinary Therapy XII*. Philadelphia: W.B. Saunders, 1995: 1365–1369.

8. Gratzek, J.B. *Aquariology: The Science of Fish Health Management*. Morris Plains, NJ: Tetra Press, 1992: 232.

9. Stoskopf, M.K. "Clinical Pathology." In Stoskopf, M.K. ed., *Fish Medicine*. Philadelphia. W.B. Saunders, 1993: 113–131.

10. Dunbar, C.E. and Wolf, K. "The Cytological Course of Experimental Lymphocystis in the Bluegill," *Journal of Infectious Disease* 116 (1996) 466–472.

11. Nemetz, T.G. and Shotts, E.B. "Zoonotic Diseases." In Stoskopf, M.K. ed., *Fish Medicine*. Philadelphia: W.B. Saunders, 1993: 214–220.